THE NEW HEART HEALTH

Discover the Power of the Endothelium

Dr. Louis Ignarro
Nobel Laureate in Medicine
&
Dr. Andrew Myers

The New Heart Health

Discover the Power of the Endothelium

by Louis Ignarro, PhD and Andrew Myers, ND

Published by
Health Value Publications

Cover and interior design: Fusion Creative Works

Primary editor and content developer: Stacy Ennis

International Standard Book Number 9781613890066

Warning-Disclaimer

Health Value Publications and Drs. Ignarro and Myers have designed this book to provide information in regard to the subject matter covered. It is sold with the understanding that the publisher and author are not liable for the misconception or misuse of information provided. Every effort has been made to make this book as complete and accurate as possible. The purpose of this book is to educate. The authors and Health Value Publications shall have neither liability nor responsibility to any person or entity with respect to loss, damage, or injury caused or alleged to be caused directly or indirectly by the information contained in this book. The information presented herein is in no way intended as a substitute for medical counseling. It is recommended that you do not self-diagnose. Proper medical care is critical to good health. If you have symptoms suggestive of an illness, please consult a physician—preferably a naturopath, holistic physician, osteopath, chiropractor, or other natural health care specialist. If you are currently taking a prescription medication, you absolutely must consult your doctor before discontinuing it.

The Nobel Foundation has no affiliation with the authors in regards to this book and has not reviewed, approved, or endorsed the content of *The New Heart Health.*

For more information, visit HealthIsWealth.net.

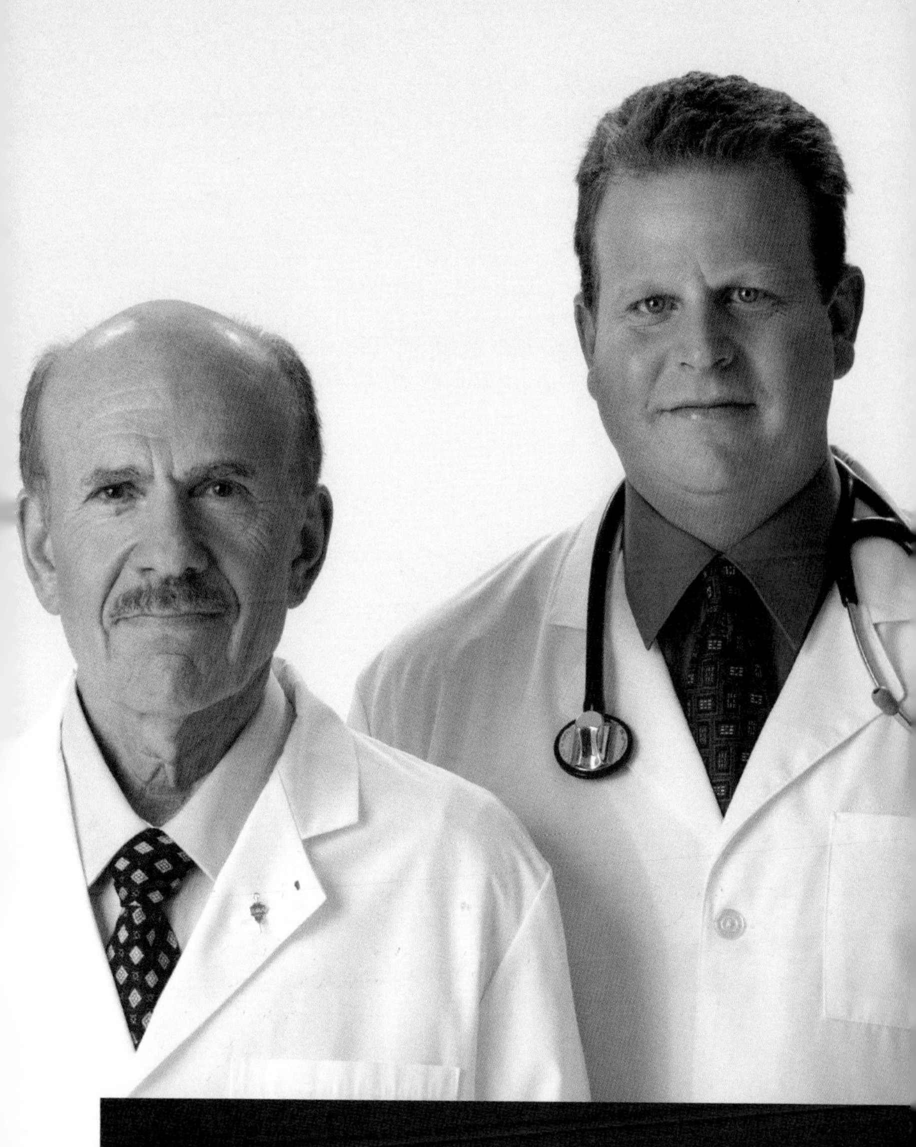

We dedicate this book to everyone who is excited about maintaining endothelial health through healthy lifestyle, and to our families and friends for their love and support.

Contents

Introduction

A Deeper Story to NO by Dr. Louis Ignarro

You are in control of your own destiny.

Thinking of "choice" and "health" as being intimately connected might seem contradictory. But it's not. You can choose to live a vital, full life free from disease. It doesn't matter how unhealthy you are today. The moment you begin changing those bad habits for good, you immediately start on the path toward health. There's always hope. No matter what else you take away from my message, I want that to resound with you.

While this is true throughout the entire body, it's especially true in the cardiovascular system. A study of more than 30,000 subjects in fifty-two countries found that over 90 percent of cardiovascular disease (CVD) is preventable through positive lifestyle changes. I'll modify that slightly: over 90 percent of CVD is preventable. That means that those little choices you make every day determine whether you will be overweight, sick, tired, and suffering cardiovascular dysfunction or fit, healthy, and energized in every system of your body. Your decisions can save you or kill you. But even if you've spent forty or more years walking down the path of heart disease, you can turn around and walk the other way. Every step you take in the opposite direction, on the road of cardiovascular health, initiates the process of reversing damage and healing your cardiovascular system.

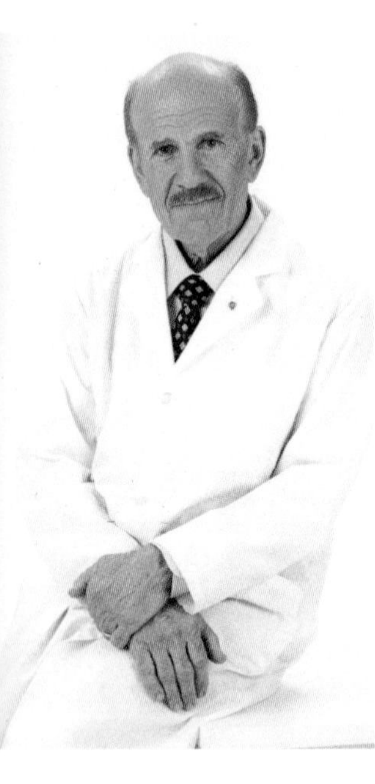

Since I'm a research pharmacologist, you might assume that I'm about to sell you on the latest cardiovascular drug. I'm not. Actually, there is no pill or capsule that can prevent or reverse CVD. A holistic approach—natural preventive medicine that treats the body, mind, and spirit as one—is the way your cardiovascular system can stay fit and healthy well into your final decades. And the scientific community is just starting to understand that the best way to approach prevention is through supplementing the body's own self-healing process.

Science works like this: researchers choose a specific focus of study, and they stay within the parameters of their subject for years, sometimes decades. In my case, it was the powerful signaling molecule nitric oxide, or NO. I studied that one tiny molecule for forty years! When my colleagues and I discovered the power of NO and were awarded the Nobel Prize in Physiology or Medicine, NO essentially became "molecule of the year." It was an exciting time for me. At the same time, thousands of scientists around the world were researching other components of the body, many with a narrow, specific area of study like me.

This focused approach is great because it helps us understand distinct elements of the body at a very deep level. But it's also troublesome because, while all of this research is going on, researchers are isolated and aren't communicating with each other. Yes, studies get published, but there are over 24,000 reputable scientific journals around the world! Each of those journals puts out dozens to hundreds of articles per year. The likelihood that two researchers will connect, share critical information, and help each other make life-altering discoveries is very, very slim. Science is a process in which individual findings feed a larger concept of health on a global scale. And for that larger concept to come together, all of the discoveries must also coalesce.

In many ways, it's like a multipiece jigsaw puzzle. Each researcher is busy exploring his tiny piece of the puzzle, but it's when all the pieces connect that great discoveries are made, ones that are useful for the general population… discoveries that can save lives.

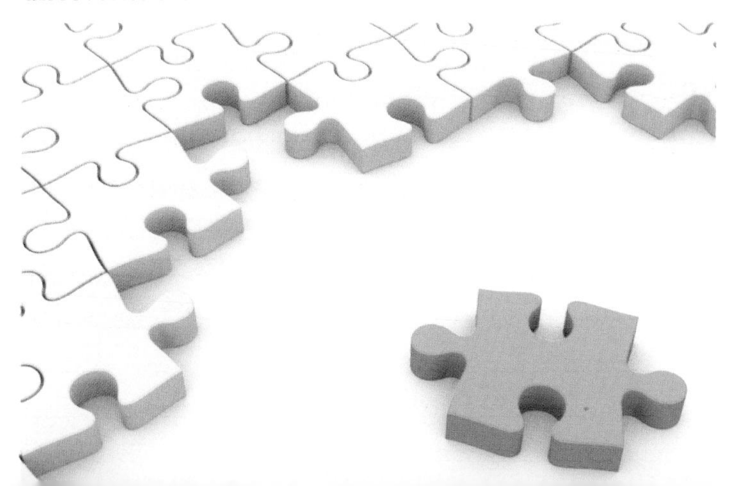

I'm not focusing on my puzzle piece anymore. I've retired from research, stepped out of the lab, and am able to see the big picture. I now review scientific studies in an effort to piece together research, both my own and from other scientists. And understanding the "cardiovascular puzzle" starts with the tiny cells that produce NO.

The scientific community is just starting to understand that the best way to approach prevention is through supplementing the body's own self-healing process. The best way to support that process is through a healthy lifestyle and a targeted supplementation regimen.

More to the NO Story

There are medical conferences that last an entire week just to describe the basic functioning of the powerful signaling molecule NO, but some of the most important aspects can be explained in a few basic points. First, NO controls blood flow through every single organ in the body. Second, NO regulates blood pressure and blood cell function, which means that it keeps blood from clotting inside the body. And third, NO regulates white blood

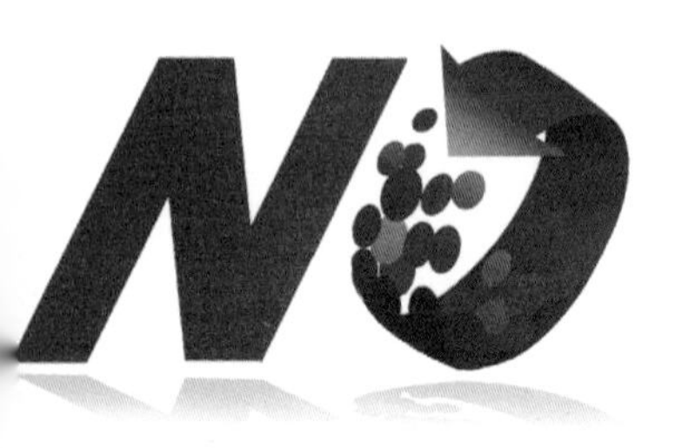

cell function. (See, "The Endothelium: Your Unknown Organ" in Section 1 for more on NO.) Those are just a few key roles of NO; there are many, many other incredible ways that NO keeps the body running smoothly. And the scientific community is continually discovering more and more about the power of this astounding molecule.

I'm a scientist. I look at things practically to figure out how they function. But this tiny molecule never fails to amaze me.

After retiring from research, I began educating people around the world about the astounding benefits of NO. As a professor at UCLA, I taught medical students about how NO functions in the cardiovascular system and its benefits throughout the entire body. As a lecturer, I've taught

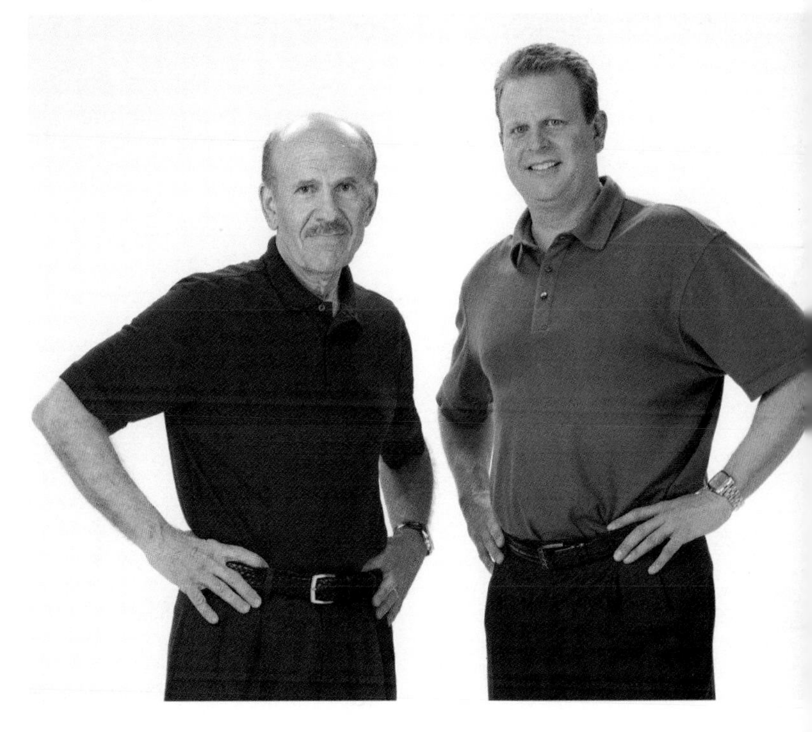

physicians and lay audiences around the world about the incredible story of NO and how to boost NO production in the body to lead to greater health and vitality.

The information I've shared has saved lives. But I now realize that there is a deeper story I need to tell. And that story starts at the cellular level.

How did I come to this realization? Well, over a decade ago, I met Dr. Andrew Myers, a naturopathic physician and expert in nutritional and herbal medicine. Dr. Myers spent months teaching me about the body's amazing self-healing properties and sharing peer-reviewed research studies that proved the importance of a healthy lifestyle. Over the years, the two of us have formed a unique partnership that combines our two areas of expertise: pharmacology and naturopathic medicine. It seems like a bit of an oxymoron, doesn't it? I specialize in prescription drugs, and he specializes in natural medicine. But, as you'll see throughout *The New Heart Health*, while we approach health from different perspectives and areas of expertise, we both arrive at the same conclusion: a holistic approach is the only answer to preventing and reversing dysfunction in the body.

As I began to embrace preventive medicine, I realized that I could apply the same concept to the cardiovascular system. I'd been looking so closely at NO for so long, zeroed in at the molecular level, that once I quit doing my own research in the lab, started examining other research studies, and learned more about naturopathic medicine, I saw a clear answer to cardiovascular dysfunction. Since NO keeps the cardiovascular system healthy, I should be focusing my studies on the organ in the body that *makes*

NO. In effect, I needed to look at a more complete picture of cardiovascular health.

This realization led me to shift my focus from one specific molecule to a system of cells. Our bodies contain six trillion endothelial cells that line one hundred thousand miles of blood vessels in a continuous, single layer. Together, those cells make up an organ known as the endothelium. Endothelial cells are the *only* cells in the arteries and veins that make NO. If your endothelium is healthy, your body will be flooded with NO. If your endothelium is unhealthy, NO levels will drop, and your cardiovascular system will become more and more dysfunctional. What follows? Heart attack, stroke, and other serious CVDs.

Endothelial dysfunction is the starting point of almost all cardiovascular dysfunction.

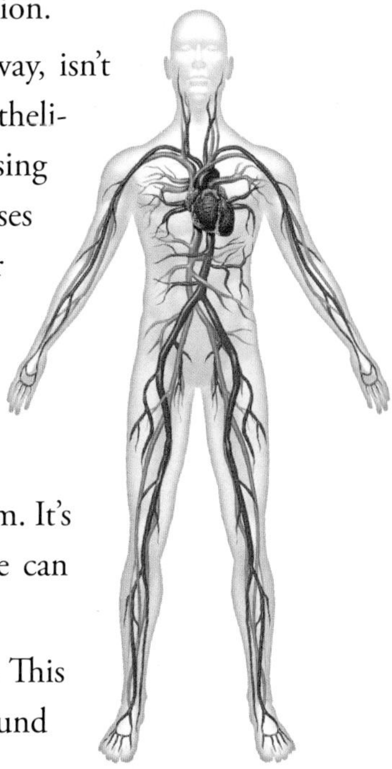

When you think about it that way, isn't it a no-brainer that a healthy endothelium is the key to preventing or reversing heart attack, stroke, and other diseases of the cardiovascular system? Your body must make enough of the lifesaving signaling molecule and antioxidant NO to function optimally. A healthy endothelium equals a healthy cardiovascular system. It's a radical concept, but one I believe can save lives around the world.

I now have a new story to share. This book is my way of helping people around the world change how they look at heart disease. Heart attack and stroke don't just strike from nowhere, like a bolt of lightning. Rather, it's a slow process of damage over many years, much like eroding soil that eventually gives way to a landslide. That damage begins with the endothelium. Similarly, the endothelium is the starting point for preventing and reversing CVD. And Dr. Myers and I will add that endothelial dysfunction is the starting point to obesity, Type 2 diabetes, and metabolic syndrome, which are all issues that lead to CVD.

The story of endothelial health is a story of empowerment. Understanding how the endothelium works puts the power back in your hands—it helps you understand how to take steps *now* to have a healthy cardiovascular system *later*.

My life's mission is to eradicate CVD by teaching the importance of endothelial health to people around the world. The mission starts with you, and each person you share the story with multiplies the effect. Someday, I believe we can accomplish this grand mission together.

Endothelial dysfunction is the starting point of almost all cardiovascular disease.

A Natural Approach by Dr. Andrew Myers

Scientific studies are absolutely necessary to helping advance what we know about the human body. But here's what's interesting about science: The body doesn't care about research, conclusive findings, or double-blind placebo-controlled studies. Science is the process by which humankind learns about something that's already perfect, already functioning, and doesn't need to understand itself to work.

As a naturopathic physician, my focus is on understanding how the human body works and finding natural ways to encourage a dysfunctional body to self-heal. Naturopathic medicine is much different than "conventional" medicine—the medical approach most of us are familiar with—in two ways. First, it treats causes, not symptoms. Second, it understands that the body, mind, and spirit cannot be separated. Let me explain what I mean.

Conventional medicine is about symptom management. If you go to a conventional doctor because you've been feeling tired and fatigued, what happens? Most likely, your doctor will ask a series of symptom-related questions, run diagnostic tests, and prescribe a drug to help alleviate the symptoms. The issue is that the symptoms aren't the problem. The dysfunction that's creating the symptoms is the problem.

Very few doctors will ask questions such as: What is your diet like? How often do you exercise? How much sleep are you getting each night? How much water are you drinking every day? Are you under emotional strain right

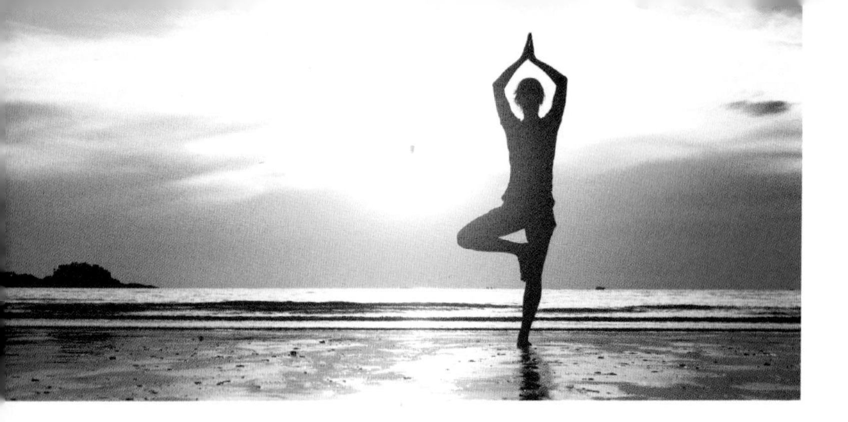

now? Instead, they poke you with needles, look at charts, and tell you to pop a pill.

But the body, mind, and spirit are all interrelated. Ignoring a person's lifestyle is the wrong way to approach wellness. Stress, for example, can be debilitating. Study after study has shown the tremendous amount of harm stress can do to the body. But, when the effects of stress result in physical symptoms like depression or chronic fatigue, what happens? I can almost guarantee conventional doctors aren't writing prescriptions for meditation, yoga, massage, or other stress-relieving activities.

Part of the Hippocratic oath, the ethical guidelines most doctors follow, says, "I will use those dietary regimens which will benefit my patients according to my greatest ability and judgment, and I will do no harm or injustice to them." Yet conventional medicine rarely looks at diet and lifestyle first, and some of the medications doctors dole out to patients are filled with toxic substances that may lead to people's demise.

I'm not suggesting that conventional medicine doesn't have its merits. If I get in a devastating car accident, I want to be taken to the emergency room, where doctors have access to lifesaving pharmaceuticals, equipment, and procedures. But if we can reframe the way we see medicine as a society, and begin to see naturopathic medicine and conventional medicine as complementary to each other, then we're starting to take an approach that can not only save lives but also help people live longer, fuller, happier lives, too.

Conventional medicine and prescription drugs aren't the only issues, and they're not the only answers, either. The high-fat, low-movement, high-stress, poor-sleep Western lifestyle has been exported to countries around the world, bringing with it a myriad of problems that are wrecking bodies globally. Cardiovascular disease is the leading cause of death around the world not because more people are being born with genetic abnormalities but because their poor lifestyle habits are literally killing them.

People don't die of heart attacks and stroke. They die because they've been starving their cardiovascular systems of critical nutrients for decades, which leads to heart attacks and stroke. There are some exceptions to this; less than 10 percent of CVD is due to unavoidable causes like injury or genetic abnormality. In general, however, most people who suffer from CVD are really suffering from Nutrient Deficiency Syndrome, or NDS (see page 65).

NDS can affect any part of the body. It occurs in the cardiovascular system when the heart, arteries, capillaries, and veins aren't getting the nutrients they need to function optimally. The starting point of cardiovascular deficiency? The endothelium. As the years go on, the cardiovascular system gets more and more deficient, until it eventually exhibits symptoms that a doctor diagnoses as CVD.

There is a better way: preventive medicine. You can optimize your cardiovascular health by using supplemental nutrition (such as vitamins and minerals) to replenish vital elements that are constantly being depleted by today's modern lifestyle. In this book, Dr. Ignarro and I will teach you strategies that can *almost guarantee* you will never have a heart attack or stroke. If you already have CVD, we'll show you how you can reverse your condition.

There is no pill that can fix your cardiovascular system. But, by taking a holistic approach to your well-being, including healthy diet, exercise, plenty of sleep, stress reduction, and supplementation, you can heal your heart, arteries, capillaries, and veins. And, as we've mentioned, that all starts with six trillion tiny cells known as the endothelium that line 100,000 miles of blood vessels in your body.

You have ultimate power over how healthy you are and how good you feel. Dr. Ignarro and I will teach you how to take control of your cardiovascular health.

The human body is already perfect, already functioning, and doesn't need to understand itself to work. Science simply gives us a window into its intricate processes.

Endothelial Health is Cardiovascular Wealth

If you've read *Health Is Wealth*, you've been introduced to the powerful analogy between health and wealth. (If you haven't read it, don't worry; I'll summarize it for you here.) I'd like to take that concept a step further: endothelial health is cardiovascular wealth.

The health is wealth concept is twofold. When you're not healthy, you aren't able to enjoy the wealth of wellness in your life. Health, to a degree, is freedom. If you're fit, well rested, getting all of your key nutrients (including the critical "10 Power Nutrients" for total wellness identified in *Health Is Wealth*), and have low stress levels, you're able to live life more fully than someone who is overweight, tired, suffering from NDS, and stressed out. That's one part of the health is wealth concept.

> Preventive medicine optimizes cardiovascular health by using supplemental nutrition (vitamins and minerals) to replenish vital elements that are constantly being depleted by today's modern lifestyle.

There's a much more practical and pragmatic element to the metaphor, though: it costs a lot more to be sick than it does to be healthy. I'm not just talking on an individual basis; it costs more on a national scale, too. The United States spends more on health care than other developed countries—double the median amount, in fact—without a marked difference in quality of care.

Health Is Wealth offers practical strategies for approaching wellness—and restoring wealth—from a total-body focus. *The New Heart Health* takes a much more focused approach by looking specifically at the endothelium. It's meant to educate and enable, to change viewpoints and inspire people toward action, with the mission of completely eradicating heart disease around the world.

Dr. Ignarro talked about our unique approach—a pharmacologist and a naturopathic physician working together—and I'd like to briefly touch on that as well. What I find remarkable about our partnership is that while I'm a generalist who understands health at a total-body level, Dr. Ignarro is a specialist in NO and the endothelium. Partnering with him has given me so much insight into the intricate functioning of the body at a molecular level. After all, he studied one tiny molecule for *forty years*. He knows the cardiovascular system in such detail that he's almost encyclopedic with his knowledge. It's incredible. There's likely no individual who knows more about the cardiovascular system than Dr. Ignarro. Having a conversation with him is like tapping into the most in-depth information resource in the world when it comes to cardiovascular health and

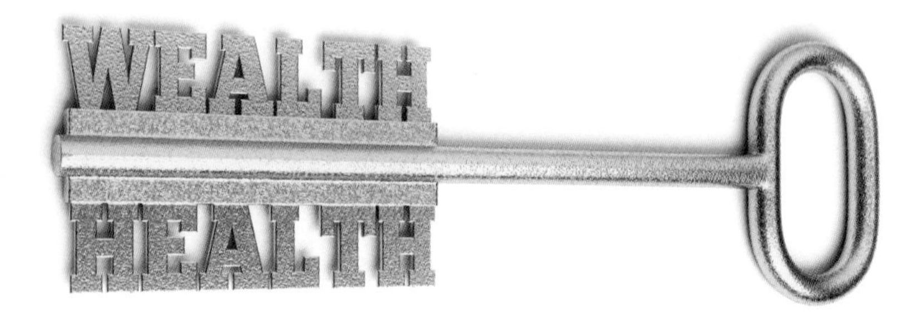

NO. We share some of that specialized information in this book. Combining our expertise, we'll teach you how to optimize your cardiovascular system by using supplemental nutrition to replenish vital elements that are constantly being depleted by today's modern lifestyle.

The human body is incredibly complex. Scientists still have so much to learn about it, and there are still many mysteries to be understood. But we do know one thing about the cardiovascular system: all dysfunction starts with the endothelial cells. By sharing the story of the endothelium, and learning how to support the restorative powers of the individual cells, Dr. Ignarro and I believe you can not only get healthy yourself, but you can also become an ambassador for heart health. People deserve a choice and chance to be well.

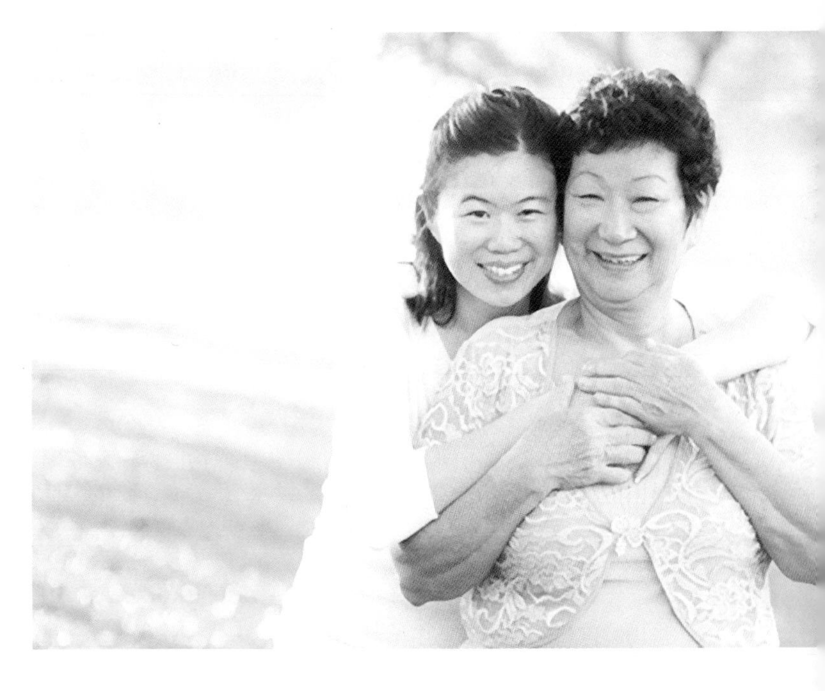

It's estimated that people spend 50 percent of their entire lifetime health expenditures in the last two weeks of their lives. A proactive, holistic approach helps avoid such expenses by focusing on health in the long-term, rather than trying to make up for decades of damage through expensive life-saving procedures.

How to Use This Book

We—Dr. Ignarro and Dr. Myers—are constantly surprised by how many cardiologists don't know about the endothelium—information about this incredible organ is *that* new. Cardiologists are supposed to be experts on the cardiovascular system, but many just don't have the time or energy to keep up with the latest research. Each year, more and more studies are conducted to understand the endothelial cells and their role in the entire body. While we don't have conclusive findings about how it affects organs like the brain, study upon study has proven the power of the endothelium in the cardiovascular system.

The New Heart Health is meant to help you understand how to keep your endothelial cells healthy and your cardiovascular system functioning optimally, well into old age. Section 1 provides an overview of what the endothelium is, how it functions, its role in the cardiovascular system, and how a healthy endothelium supports cardiovascular health. Section 2 explains how endothelial dysfunction is the starting point for what most doctors diagnose as CVD and breaks down factors that can cause endothelial cells to become dysfunctional. Section 3 is the "solutions" chapter, which will help you create a targeted lifestyle and supplementation regimen to get your endothelium healthy and functioning at its peak. We've also included a detailed overview of 10 Power Nutrients for endothelial health in Section 3 that anyone can combine with a healthy lifestyle to help prevent and reverse heart disease. Finally, you'll find full-color images throughout the book that further explain specific concepts. Consider *The New Heart Health* a guide to a topic that will be a major focus of cardiovascular medicine going forward. You'll learn information in these pages that some cardiovascular specialists don't even know.

Scan this QR code with your smartphone to access healthiswealth.net

As part of this educational project, we've also created a library of resources on our website, HealthIsWealth.net. It's a continually growing site that covers the latest health information in an easy-to-understand, engaging format. You can find more about heart health and total bodily wellness on our site, as well as free resources like downloadable PDFs detailing the Power Nutrients in Section 3 of this book.

Our number one goal for both this book and our website is to offer education that you can use and share. Whether you're twenty-five and forming your lifelong habits or sixty-seven and getting healthy after a first heart attack, we offer critical information that can impact your life for the better.

Your life span is directly related to the health of your cells. The healthier your cells, the longer you'll live and the more vital you'll be as you age. A preventive approach is best when started early because damage done to the body is cumulative. But the amazing thing about the endothelium—the story we're so excited to share—is that anyone, at any time, at any level of health, can reverse CVD. Anyone. And that includes you.

By learning how the endothelium works, you begin to understand that you have a choice. You can choose health. We offer you the information and tools you need to take the first step in changing your life.

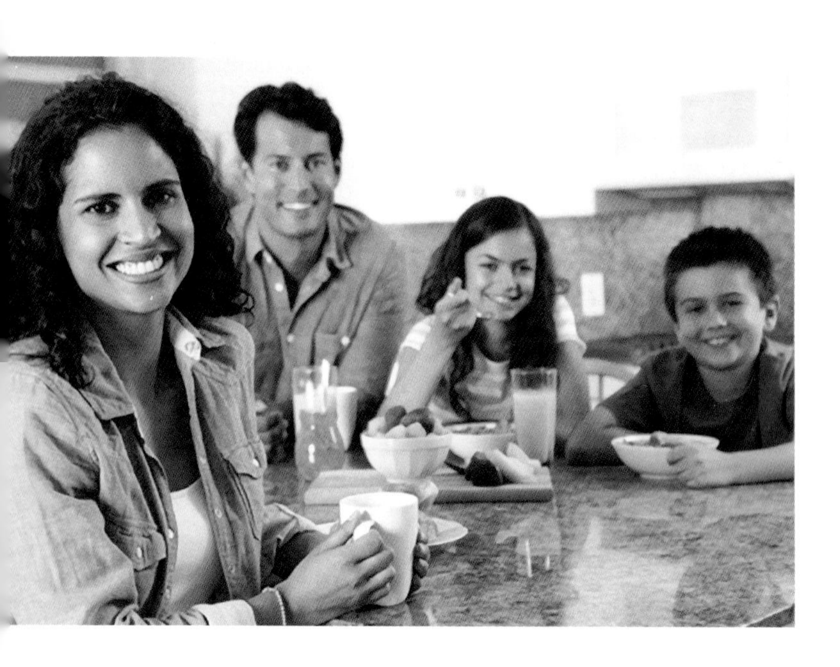

Section 1

The Endothelium: Your Unknown Organ

What have you done today? Aside from the intentional movement you make throughout the day—standing up to greet someone, scratching an itch on your arm, waving hello to a friend—you have very little control over the bulk of the functioning of your body. While you were going about your daily activities, your body was regulating processes you didn't even have to think about. In fact, most of your movement throughout the day is reflexive, meaning some of your muscles function without your conscious involvement.

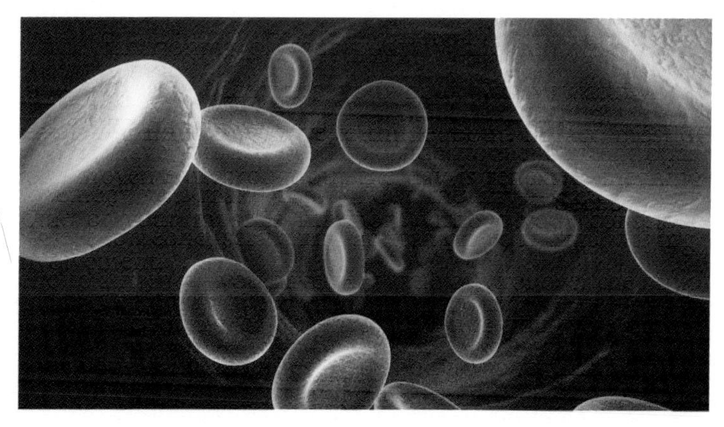

Your heart is one such muscle. It pumps about five quarts of blood per minute through the arteries, veins, and capillaries without so much as a thought from you. It nourishes the organs and tissues of the body, adjusts to meet the demands you place on it, and beats about one hundred thousand times per day to keep your entire body functioning—even while you sleep.

But have you ever stopped to wonder *how* the heart does all of this, day after day, without rest? On top of that, how does the blood flow efficiently through the various components of the cardiovascular system? All of these processes depend on an almost unknown organ: the endothelium.

Looking at the Big Picture: The Cardiovascular Story

We can't go a page further without explaining how the health of this almost unknown organ, the endothelium, relates to the bigger story of cardiovascular health. You see, endothelial cells are absolutely critical to the function of the heart, arteries, veins, and capillaries, and the prevention or reversal of heart disease. At its most basic level, the endothelium is the foundation of the entire cardiovascular system. That's a powerful statement, but a true one.

In the conventional medical system, researchers and physicians like to talk about the various components of the cardiovascular system—from the heart down to the capillaries—and address disease as it relates to those isolated parts. If you go in for a checkup, your doctor will probably discuss plaque buildup, platelet stickiness, cholesterol levels, blood pressure levels...basically all of the states that reflect how well your cardiovascular system is functioning. But we've found that a broader approach is to focus on the health of the endothelium. Endothelial health is the baseline by which the entire cardiovascular system can be evaluated, since each and every cardiovascular component is impacted by the endothelium.

Unfortunately, people around the world aren't taking the needed steps to support endothelial health. Just as a healthy endothelium means a healthy cardiovascular system, an unhealthy endothelium can result in an unhealthy cardiovascular system. Consider the statistics:

- Cardiovascular disease (CVD) is the leading cause of death globally, not just in the Western world.
- More people die from CVD than cancer, AIDS, or any other single cause.
- Heart disease accounts for one in four deaths in the United States.
- CVD and stroke account for one-third of all female deaths globally.
- More women die of heart disease each year than men in the United States.
- In the United States, someone suffers from a heart attack every thirty-four seconds.
- One person dies every minute in the United States from a cause related to heart disease.

- Less than 10 percent of cases of CVD are due to genetics, injury, or other unavoidable conditions.

These numbers provide a grim glimpse into the future of heart health. But we'd like to tell you a different story. For us, the "cardiovascular story" is really about putting the power back in your hands. Remember: 90 percent of CVD is *preventable or reversible* through healthy lifestyle changes. If everyone embraced the strategies and information in this book, we believe that heart disease statistics could be drastically reduced. Instead of 11.5 percent of Americans suffering from heart disease, what if that number could be 1 or 2 percent? How different would our country be? It's absolutely possible. But for that to happen, people must learn the critical story of how the endothelium impacts the cardiovascular system. The best way to start is understanding what the endothelium is and how it functions.

Someone suffers from a heart attack every thirty-four seconds and dies from a heart disease-related cause every minute in the United States.

What Is the Endothelium?

The endothelium is an organ system within the cardiovascular system. The cardiovascular system is made up of the heart and a system of blood vessels composed of arteries, veins, and capillaries. The arteries carry oxygen-rich blood (thanks to oxygen from the lungs) from the heart to the rest of the organs and tissues in the body through tiny capillaries, which release the oxygen to the cells and take up carbon dioxide. Blood then flows from the capillaries into the veins and travels back to the heart to be reoxygenated. This entire process takes about a minute, depending on how active you are; the more you move, the faster your blood flows.

Here's where the endothelium comes in. Your body contains six trillion endothelial cells that line one hundred thousand miles of blood vessels in a single layer; that continuous layer throughout the vascular system (the arteries, veins, and capillaries) makes up the endothelium. The main job of the endothelium is to create the signaling molecule nitric oxide (NO), the most important molecule in the entire cardiovascular system.

The endothelium extends throughout the entire body but has different functions in different parts of the body. Endothelial cells function differently in the brain, for example, than in the liver, kidney, or lungs. But that's another topic and another book—for now, we'll focus on its role in the cardiovascular system.

We mentioned that the endothelium is a component of the cardiovascular system but also a separate organ. Because endothelial cells form a communicative layer—one touching another throughout the entire body—they're considered a single entity. This shakes up what most people know about organs. After all, what do you think of when you hear the word "organ"? The liver, the lungs, the heart—basically, a singular mass within the body that you could put your hands around. The research community even used to think the endothelium was simply a protective layer within the blood vessels. It took decades for scientists to finally recognize that the endothelium is a communicative layer of cells, one organ that has its own unique function within the body. And, as it turns out, the organ also has one of the most important roles in the cardiovascular system.

Why are the endothelial cells so important? Along with helping to regulate blood flow, the endothelium is the factory that produces and releases NO and a handful of other hormones and chemicals that influence all aspects of cardiovascular health.

Actually, you could even say the endothelium is life-giving. During the fetal period, the vascular system, lined with the endothelium, is one of the first developments in a growing baby. The blood vessels are necessary to the development of the fetus because blood provides the nutrition and oxygen—basically everything a developing human needs to grow—and removes the cellular toxins and waste out of the body.

As a fetus grows, it needs more blood vessels to build new tissues. The endothelium expands and generates more cells and drives the development of adjacent organs. NO facilitates this process with the endothelium at the root of it all. The endothelial cells are directly related to the progression of development and growth; without them, developing babies wouldn't be able to survive. Without your endothelium, you wouldn't be here.

Some scientists even think that understanding how endothelial cells communicate during fetal development might help us understand more about diseases like diabetes and cancer. That's what's so exciting about the endothelium—we already know it's a powerful organ, but there are more and more health secrets being uncovered all the time.

The endothelium is an amazing organ. Endothelial health is linked to all organ and cell health throughout the entire body, and the endothelium is directly related to the function of every cell in the body. Isn't that incredible?

How the Endothelium Functions

Some people have described the endothelium as the Teflon inside the blood vessels because it allows the blood to flow smoothly and evenly. That's true, but it does much more. The endothelium is:

- **Protective.** The endothelium prevents toxic substances in the blood from entering the smooth muscle within the wall of the blood vessel, as well as helps keep the blood from getting sticky and forming a clot.

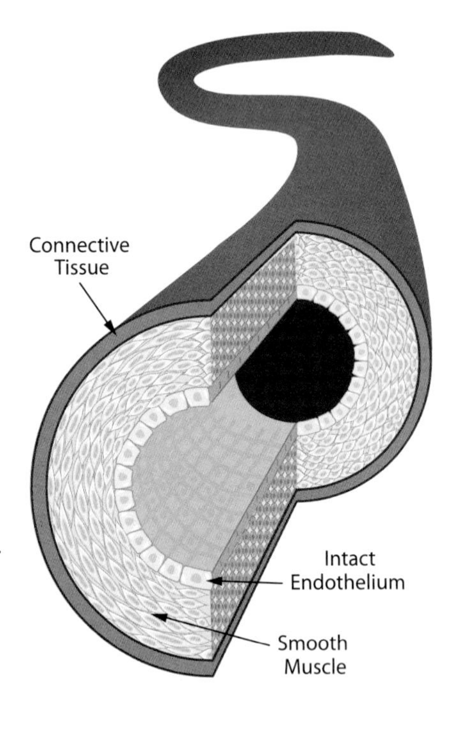

- **Secretory.** Endothelial cells secrete substances that tell the blood vessels to dilate or contract. Its major function? The production and secretion of the most important molecule in the cardiovascular system, NO.
- **Dynamic.** Blood vessels aren't just a tubing system through which blood flows. The endothelium helps the arteries and veins expand and contract to reg-

ulate blood pressure and maintain healthy blood circulation.

- **Reactive.** The endothelium reacts to the pressures placed on it—from stress, exercise, and dietary choices, among other factors—by releasing hormones and chemicals to tell the blood vessels how to deal with those pressures.
- **Healing.** Most amazingly, the endothelium has the ability to self-heal. When it senses injury, it sends signals to the arterial walls that tell the arteries how to heal and can even regenerate endothelial cells.

The endothelium is highly adaptable and responsive; in many ways, it is a "super organ," nourishing the muscles, organs, and tissues and allowing the blood to flow evenly throughout the entire body. It lines each and every artery and blood vessel in the body and controls and regulates the local environment within the blood vessel.

To understand how the endothelium works, let's take a look at a diagram of an artery (see Image 1.1). You'll notice that arteries have three layers: the inner layer is the endothelium; the middle layer contains smooth muscle that expands or contracts to regulate blood flow; and the outer layer of connective tissue anchors the arteries to surrounding tissue. As blood flows over the endothelial cells, it stimulates the endothelium to release hormones, chemicals, and other substances to help regulate blood flow and provide other necessary benefits to the cardiovascular system.

The endothelium's main function is the secretion of NO, the molecule that signals the middle layer of smooth muscle to expand or contract in response to pressures placed on the arteries. NO is released both "inward" into the smooth muscle wall and "outward" into the circulating blood. (NO has several other functions in the cardiovascular system; see page 42 for more.) As a protective layer, the endothelium also keeps toxic substances out of the smooth muscle arterial wall so the middle layer can do its job.

Since arteries carry blood away from the heart, they're the blood vessels that also receive the full impact of each heartbeat. So, while the health of the veins and capillaries is important, the arteries tend to have the most pressure placed on them. That's why it's necessary for the arteries to be smooth and flexible so they can respond to changes in blood flow. If you're sitting, stand up. What did you notice? Probably not much. That's because your endothelium sent out hormones, chemicals, and other substances to adjust the blood flow in your body as you changed positions. Your endothelial cells react almost instantaneously—so fast, in fact, that you likely didn't sense any change in your body. Imagine if every time you stood up, you got lightheaded, felt dizzy, and fell over! That wouldn't just be a pain; it would make it nearly impossible to function. Thankfully, as you move, your endothelium responds by sending signals that contract certain blood vessels and expand others, so your blood can flow effectively, and you can go about your day-to-day activities.

In addition to maintaining blood flow, your endothelium also helps keep your blood from getting sticky. Now, your blood needs to become sticky in certain circumstances—for example, when you have a cut, your blood platelets stick together and form a clot to stop the bleeding. In that case, sticking and clotting is a good thing. But when the blood *itself* becomes too sticky—without a trigger, like a cut—it can result in platelet aggregation, a condition in which blood platelets can stick to the walls of arteries. This can lead to blood clots, which cause heart attack and stroke. When your endothelium is healthy, it produces plenty of NO, the critical signaling molecule that helps reduce inflammation in the blood vessel walls and prevent platelet aggregation.

The endothelial cells also help control blood pressure. The term "blood pressure" is used so frequently that it's easy to overlook what it *is*, exactly. It's actually pretty simple: blood pressure is the pressure placed on the arteries as blood flows through them. The less flexible your arteries are, the harder the force against the arterial wall as blood moves through the vessels. Plaque buildup, sticky blood, inflammation—all of these make it harder for the blood to flow efficiently. That means your heart has to work harder to pump your blood, which puts more strain on the heart. When the endothelium is healthy, it releases NO, which helps keep the blood vessels flexible, reduces inflammation, and causes the blood vessels to dilate, among other benefits.

Most of us have tried to blow up a long, thin balloon before—the kind balloon artists use to make animals and funny hats for children. If you take one right out of the bag, put it to your mouth, and attempt to blow it up, not much happens. Considering the balloon as a blood vessel and your breath as blood is a good analogy for a dysfunctional vessel. It's incredibly difficult for blood to flow through a nearly closed, rigid vessel. But if you manually stretch the balloon with your hands to open it up and make it more elastic and flexible, and then attempt to blow it up again, what occurs? The balloon easily inflates. Similarly, a healthy endothelium helps the blood vessel maintain elasticity and relaxes the muscular layer so the vessel can stretch to accommodate and respond to blood flow and pressure. The presence of NO causes the vessel to relax and tighten itself as needed. And this all happens because of the amazing endothelium!

When your endothelium is healthy, it's your biggest ally in preventing diseases like atherosclerosis (hardening of the arteries), inflammation (which can lead to heart disease), and a number of other conditions. It really is a super organ, isn't it?

The endothelium is highly adaptable and responsive; in many ways, it's a "super organ," nourishing the muscles, organs, and tissues and allowing the blood to flow evenly throughout the entire body.

Case Study: Kim and the Healthy Endothelium

We think the best way to understand how the endothelium works is to "see" it in action. Meet our fictional study subject, Kim. A thirty-eight-year-old female, Kim leads a healthy lifestyle. She gets eight hours of sleep most nights; exercises five days a week; practices yoga to help lower her stress levels; maintains a healthy weight; eats a healthy diet rich in protein, low-fat dairy, whole grains, and fresh fruits and vegetables; and takes supplements to fill in the nutritional gaps that inevitably occur in her diet.

We'll start with Kim's morning routine. She wakes up at 6:00 a.m. after a full night's sleep and starts her day with a protein shake and fresh fruit. This nutritional boost helps kick-start her endothelium and gives the endothelial cells the nutrients they need to function optimally throughout the day.

Kim then heads out for a forty-minute run. Movement stimulates her endothelial cells by increasing blood flow and putting "shear stress" on her blood vessels (see page 88 for more on shear stress). As blood flows over the endothelial cells, stretching the endothelium, the cells come to life and produce NO. Not only that, but because blood flow is at its maximum, and NO levels are high, oxygen and nutrients are more effectively delivered to her exercising muscles. The best part is that Kim is not just increasing NO production during her workout; since she exercises regularly, her endothelial cells will continuously produce more NO all day long. The more she moves, the healthier her endothelium is because it's being bathed by NO, oxygen, and other nutrients—all benefits of enhanced blood flow. It's a synergistic effect.

On the outside, Kim looks healthy and fit. On the inside, she is healthy and fit, too. Her blood vessels are smooth and flexible and dilate or expand as needed, she doesn't have plaque buildup on her vessel walls, and her blood flows smoothly and isn't sticky. Her blood pressure levels are within healthy range, so her heart isn't working harder than it needs to.

One day, Kim has to work through her lunch hour and decides to pick up fast food: a hamburger and fries. This is a rare occurrence for Kim. As she eats this unhealthy meal, her healthy endothelium keeps her vessels under continual surveillance, assessing conditions like: Does the blood seem too sticky? Is it too thick? Is there too much pressure on the vessel walls? Since her endothelium is healthy, her cardiovascular system is able to adjust and respond to this once-in-a-while meal. Instead of the saturated fats damaging her endothelial cells, her endothelium is able to produce more hormones, chemicals, and other substances to deal with the influx of unhealthy food.

Kim proactively supports endothelial health through living a healthy lifestyle. By making great choices most of the time, she supports the health of her cardiovascular system day and night, even when she makes not-so-great choices.

No one is perfect, and it's nearly impossible to choose perfect nutrition all the time. But, just like Kim, by keeping your endothelium as healthy as possible, you, too, can help counteract some of the negative effects those imperfect choices have on your cardiovascular system.

Keeping your endothelium healthy allows your cardiovascular system to adjust and respond to the various pressures placed on it throughout the day.

NO: The Most Important Molecule for Cardiovascular Health

We've talked about how the endothelium is the major producer of NO, the most important molecule and powerful antioxidant in the cardiovascular system. To recap: the healthier your endothelium, the more NO is produced, and the healthier your cardiovascular system will be.

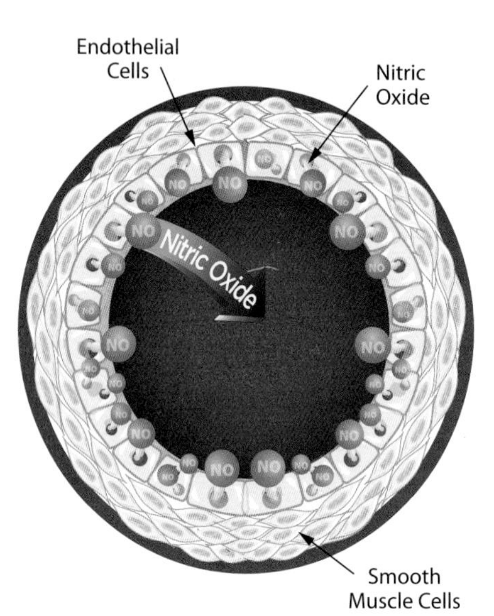

NO is an unstable, short-lived gas that is naturally produced by the body. By "short-lived," we mean it has a lifespan of less than one second. That's partially why it took so long for Dr. Ignarro and his colleagues to understand the amazing effects of this critical molecule. We are still learning about NO, but what we do know is absolutely remarkable. As a signaling molecule in the cardiovascular system, NO:

- Is a vasodilator for the arteries and veins, which means it causes the blood vessels to expand. This results in healthy blood pressure levels.

- Increases local blood flow and delivery of oxygen and nutrients to vital organs, especially the skeletal muscle.

- Keeps the blood from getting sticky, which helps prevent platelet aggregation and blood clots, thereby lowering the incidence of heart attack and stroke.
- Is an antioxidant and is anti-inflammatory, which helps prevent CVD, including heart attack and stroke.
- Aids in the prevention and treatment of coronary artery disease and atherosclerosis, or hardening of the arteries.

Here's what you really need to know: healthy endothelial cells produce ample NO, which leads to a healthy cardiovascular system.

You've now learned what the endothelium is and how a healthy endothelium keeps the cardiovascular system functioning at its best. The greatest part? You now have information many cardiologists don't even know. In Section 2, we'll explore endothelial dysfunction: what it is and what causes it. Then, we'll share some news in Section 3 that might just save your life.

When your endothelial cells are healthy, they produce ample NO, which leads to a healthy cardiovascular system.

Section 2
Endothelial Dysfunction

Think of your endothelial cells as tiny light bulbs lining a system of flexible tubes. The bulbs are glowing brilliantly because they're receiving exactly what they need to stay healthy: good nutrition and water intake, plenty of exercise, lots of sleep, and low stress levels. If you look down one tube, you'll see all of the bulbs brightly lit, the light forming a protective barrier that keeps the tubes—your blood vessels—from getting damaged. That's a healthy endothelium.

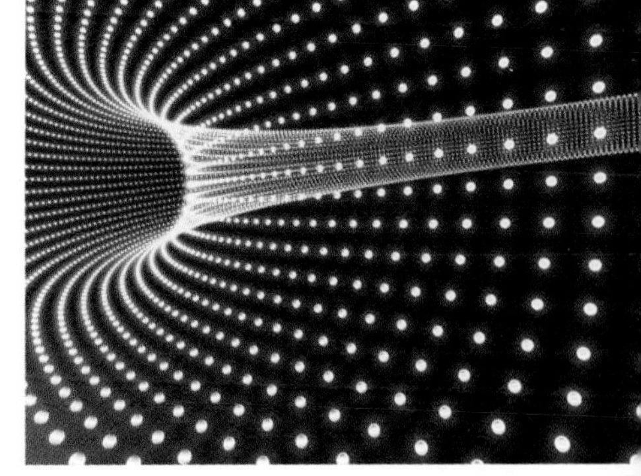

But, over time, imagine that some of the bulbs grow dim or go out completely. Poor nutrition, insufficient water intake, a sedentary lifestyle, inadequate sleep, and high stress cause the bulbs to weaken or die. Now, when you look down the tubes, you see clusters of dark spots, areas where the endothelium has been weakened. The outer tubes, the vessel walls, are now compromised because there are holes in the protective layer keeping the bad stuff out. That's endothelial dysfunction.

When cells weaken or die, it affects the wellness of the entire body. Have you ever heard Aristotle's saying, "The whole is greater than the sum of its parts"? Well, it applies to the body, too: when endothelial cells work together in full strength—as a team, a continuous layer, each doing their jobs—the entire body is healthier. But, when endothelial cells become dysfunctional, the reverse is true, and the body becomes sicker and sicker, eventually leading to multiple issues, including cardiovascular dysfunction.

We covered several of the benefits of a healthy endothelium in Section 1. Now, let's explore what endothelial dysfunction is, how it happens, and why it's so detrimental to your cardiovascular system. Then, we'll give you some good—no, great—news.

Poor nutrition, insufficient water intake, a sedentary lifestyle, inadequate sleep, and high stress can cause the individual cells that make up the endothelium to weaken and die. This compromises the vessel wall and can lead to cardiovascular disease (CVD).

Endothelial Dysfunction: The Basics

Endothelial dysfunction is a heavily researched topic, and more is learned about the endothelial cells almost every day. Endothelial dysfunction has implications in every system in the body. But there are multiple research studies proving the role of the endothelium in cardiovascular dysfunction. Simply put, endothelial dysfunction occurs when the cells of the endothelium are no longer carrying out their normal functions. In the cardiovascular system, this means the heart, arteries, veins, and capillaries aren't receiving all of the benefits we discussed in Section 1 (see page 34).

Instead of the powerful antioxidant nitric oxide (NO) flooding the cardiovascular system, NO levels fall, along with other secretory functions of the endothelium. When the dysfunctional endothelium isn't sending out chemical signals that tell the blood vessels what to do, the arteries and veins aren't able to expand, contract, and carry out the other actions they rely on the endothelium to regulate. As individual cells become dysfunctional, the endothelium's protective quality is compromised, putting the smooth muscle of the artery at risk. That's when plaque buildup and other cardiovascular risk factors occur. And plaque buildup can lead to atherosclerosis, or hardening of the arteries, which can cause a heart attack or stroke.

We talk about NO as a powerful antioxidant. The word "antioxidant" literally means "anti-oxidant," meaning it's combating the negative impact of oxidation on the body, both from internal and external sources. When the body is put under stress through poor lifestyle habits like smok-

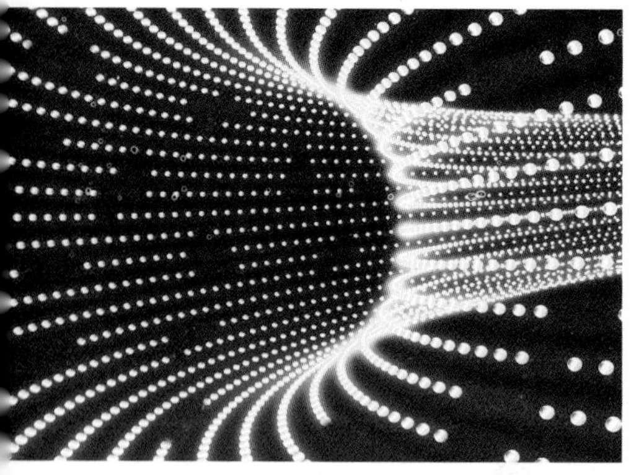

ing or chronic stress, oxidation can occur. Oxidation creates free radicals, which are unstable molecules or atoms that try to find other molecules to help them stabilize. This process disrupts the stable molecules. The body's attempt to maintain health and deal with these troublesome free radicals causes a wake of damage known as oxidative stress. Antioxidants like NO help negate the damage of free radicals.

Let's go back to our light bulb analogy. The endothelium has become weakened from a number of risk factors (we'll look at how that happens later in this section), causing the protective light bulbs (endothelial cells) lining the flexible tubes (smooth muscle arterial wall) to become dim or go out. Now that the bulbs have been damaged, pockets of the tube wall aren't protected, allowing substances in the blood like cholesterol, fats, and cellular waste to build up in the tube wall. The healthy endothelial cells, the bulbs that are still lit, send out a signal to the body to send white blood cells—known as monocytes—to travel to the area of dysfunction and light the bulbs back up. But, due to a number of chemical reactions that occur because of the damage, the white blood cells can't do their jobs. As this process is repeated over and over, the damaged white blood cells accumulate and form plaque. Plaque is an accumulation of immune cells, cellular debris that contains cholesterol and other fats, calcium, and fibrous connective tissue. The plaque continues to build up, causing the previously flexible walls of the tubes, or arteries, to thicken.

As a result of plaque buildup, cells in the tube, or the smooth muscle of the arterial wall, begin to multiply and move to the surface of the plaque, creating a firm layer and causing the tube to harden. It's no longer flexible now; if you were to try to bend or twist the tube, it would give just slightly. Looking down that tunnel of light now, you'd see that the pockets of dysfunction have grown and bulged, creating mounds of plaque. Plaque buildup limits blood flow to the organs because the walls of the tube thicken, and the inside of the tube (known as the lumen) becomes narrowed and constricted. Because of this, the volume of blood flow can become greatly restricted.

You might be aware that Dr. Ignarro's Nobel Prize-winning research on NO led to the development of Viagra, a drug that treats erectile dysfunction, or ED. While an unhealthy endothelium can cause impotence, we're focusing on the "other" ED—*endothelial* dysfunction.

As the buildup continues, those mounds can eventually erupt or break off, sending pieces of plaque into the bloodstream. The plaque particles can contribute to the formation of a blood clot, which can partially or completely block blood flow. The result? Possible heart attack or stroke.

Endothelial dysfunction occurs, even as the endothelial cells work to repair damage. But when the cells don't get a chance to self-heal, and poor lifestyle habits continue,

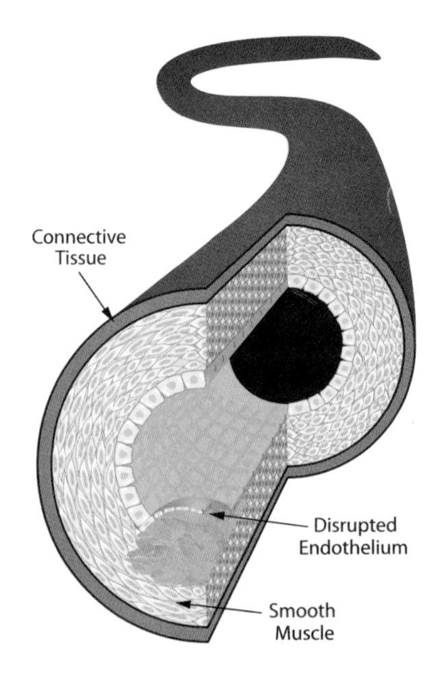

this healing mechanism actually leads to more damage. It's a dysfunctional cycle. The endothelium isn't causing the damage—it's doing what it's naturally meant to do by trying to heal. But because the body's in such a bad state, those natural processes go haywire.

Endothelial dysfunction occurs when the cells of the endothelium are no longer carrying out their normal functions.

Why Haven't I Heard of It?

The endothelium is one of the most important organs in your body and produces the most critical molecule in the cardiovascular system, NO. Endothelial dysfunction is at the root of what conventional doctors diagnose as CVD. So, why haven't you heard of endothelial dysfunction before reading this book? Moreover, why hasn't your *doctor* heard of it?

The reason is simple: there's no drug to treat it. The conditions and diseases that get attention from news media, medical organizations, and, of course, pharmaceutical companies are ones that can be "solved" with a pill, injection, surgery, or other medical intervention. Sadly, many doctors today receive their information from drug companies, rather than legitimate peer-reviewed studies that approach health holistically. "Education" surrounds prescription drugs to treat symptoms.

Preventing or reversing endothelial dysfunction involves nutrition, lifestyle, and other choices you have total control over. There is no quick-fix drug for the endothelium. That's why the companies that create and disperse information to conventional doctors—who then share information with patients like you—don't make endothelium-related research or education available.

Endothelial dysfunction can lead to atherosclerosis, or hardening of the arteries. Atherosclerosis raises the risk of heart attack or stroke. When you look at it that way, can you see how endothelial dysfunction is really one of the first steps on the dysfunctional road to CVD?

Risk Factors

Remember how we said 90 percent of CVD—really, endothelial dysfunction—is preventable or reversible through good lifestyle choices? Well, the opposite is also true: poor lifestyle choices can cause endothelial dysfunction, which eventually manifests itself as heart disease.

Leading a semi-healthy lifestyle isn't enough. Running a few miles a day, for example, won't counteract eating fast food for lunch every afternoon. Eating well and exercising won't completely negate the effects of a high-stress lifestyle or not getting enough sleep. All aspects of a healthy-heart lifestyle must be in place to keep your endothelium functioning at its peak and your cardiovascular system working smoothly.

About 37 percent of adults report two or more risk factors for heart disease. Are you one of them? Let's look at seven of the major risks for endothelial dysfunction.

Leading a semi-healthy lifestyle isn't enough. All aspects of a healthy-heart lifestyle must be in place to keep your endothelium functioning at its peak and your cardiovascular system working smoothly.

Sedentary Lifestyle

Less than half of American adults meet the Centers for Disease Control and Prevention's (CDC) physical activity recommendation of 150 minutes of exercise per week. Those are startling statistics! A sedentary lifestyle creates a higher risk of early death, depression, stroke, heart disease, Type 2 diabetes, and some cancers, not to mention endothelial dysfunction. That means that over half of US adults are much more likely to develop some type of dysfunction because they choose not to move.

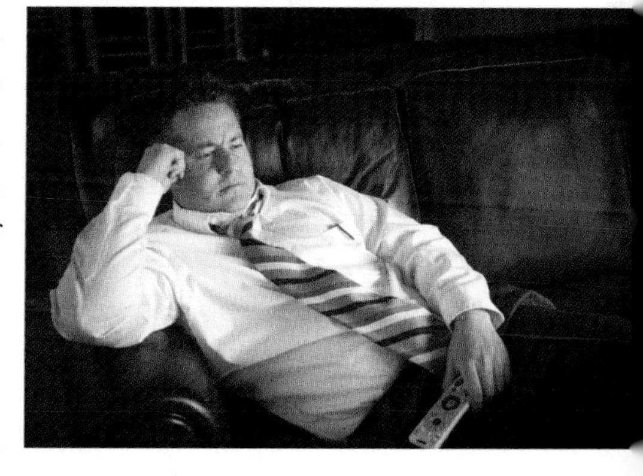

Our ancestors didn't have to exercise. They got their workouts in while hoeing the cornfields, walking to the general store, chopping wood, and even washing laundry. But we have ample opportunities to avoid movement today. From cars to escalators to washing machines, ours is a society of convenience. These conveniences are great and save us hours of work every day. But the downside is that many people aren't moving enough. A low-movement lifestyle could have a devastating impact on your endothelium.

It works like this: the less you move, the less your endothelial cells are stimulated by increased blood flow, and the less NO is produced. As you recall, NO is the most important signaling molecule in the cardiovascular system because it causes vasodilation, or the widening of blood vessels. It also acts as a powerful antioxidant, binding to the free radicals that can cause damage in the cardiovascular system. When you lead a sedentary lifestyle, your endothelium isn't able to produce enough of the critical NO your cardiovascular system needs to function at its best. Conversely, movement of any kind stimulates the endothelium and starts you on the path toward health. The moment you begin moving is the moment your endothelium starts to heal.

Poor Nutrition

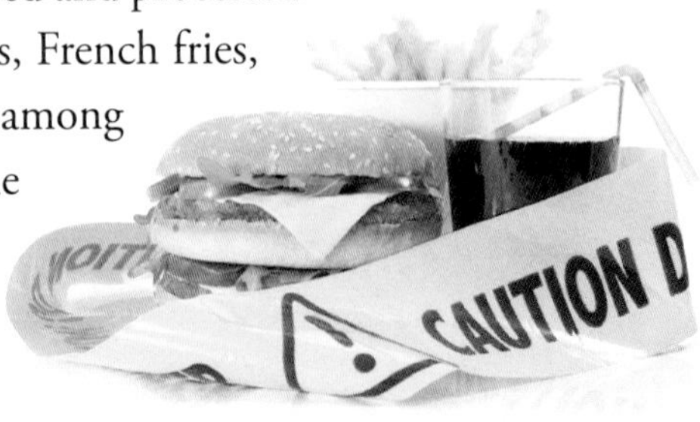

A study at Harvard School of Public Health and Channing Laboratory found that good nutrition positively impacts endothelial function. The researchers also found that eating a diet rich in fruits, vegetables, legumes, fish, poultry, and whole grains benefits the endothelial cells. But the "Western diet"—red and processed meats, sweets, desserts, French fries, and refined grains, among other staples—has the opposite effect. Not only does the poor nutrition typical of this diet rob the body of the essential nutrients it needs, it also bombards the cells with unhealthy fats, "bad" cholesterol, and excessive levels of Omega-6s. These substances can damage the individual endothelial cells and lead to plaque, inflammation, and a number of other issues.

It's important to understand that the Western diet isn't a "Western" problem. Actually, the unhealthy eating habits characteristic of Americans have spread around the globe. Even undeveloped countries have fast food readily available. People who once ate locally grown fruits, vegetables, whole grains, and meats are now indulging in high-fat, processed foods like burgers and fries…and topping that off with a chemical-laden shake or soda. These poor dietary choices are wrecking their endothelium and leading them down a path toward obesity, Type 2 diabetes, and, eventually, heart disease.

Even individuals who make relatively good dietary choices don't usually get all of the nutrients their bodies need to keep their endothelium functioning properly. That's partially because certain nutrients aren't readily available in food (vitamin D, for example). But it's also because it's incredibly hard to always get an excellent variety of vitamins and nutrients to keep your body in top form. You would have to keep close track of every morsel that crosses your lips to make sure you're getting adequate nutritional intake.

Nobody's perfect, and no one can eat a perfect diet. That's why supplementation is so important. We'll take a close look at 10 Power Nutrients to support heart health in Section 3.

> **The unhealthy eating habits characteristic of Americans have spread around the globe, making the Western diet no longer just a "Western" problem.**

Obesity

Obesity often naturally results from poor nutrition and a sedentary lifestyle. Most people know that obesity—particularly fat around the midsection—is a risk factor for CVD. Not only does it contribute to an increase in cholesterol and blood sugar levels, triglycerides, and blood pressure, but it can also lead to mood disorders like depression. It's such a serious issue that obesity is now considered a disease by the American Medical Association. But *how* does it increase risk?

Researchers used to think excess fat was just a heavy nuisance. Now, it's clear that extra fat cells release chemicals into the bloodstream that increase inflammation in the body. Inflammation erodes the endothelial lining and weakens or kills endothelial cells. Not only does this limit the secretory function of the endothelium, including the production of NO, but it also means the arterial walls are compromised. When fats, cholesterol, and other substances enter the blood stream, they have the potential to enter the arterial walls and lead to plaque buildup. (For more on how plaque forms, see "Endothelial Dysfunction: The Basics," page 47.)

More than one-third of US adults are obese, according to the CDC. Being overweight or obese damages the endothelium and significantly increases the likelihood of heart disease, stroke, Type 2 diabetes, and several types of cancers, making weight maintenance of critical importance.

The Five "Highs"

High LDL/low HDL cholesterol, high triglycerides, high insulin, high blood sugar, high blood pressure—they all tend to naturally progress from poor diet, a sedentary lifestyle, and obesity. Not surprisingly, these five "highs" are also major risk factors for endothelial dysfunction.

LDL is known as "bad" cholesterol (even though it's a lipoprotein, not cholesterol), and high LDL levels can force fat to penetrate the endothelium and contribute to plaque buildup. Oxidized LDL can also cause severe vascular damage (see page 47 for more on oxidation). On the other hand, HDL, known as "good" cholesterol (also a lipoprotein), helps clear the blood of extraneous cholesterol, helping prevent CVD. When HDL levels are low, this protective quality is compromised, and cholesterol can enter the endothelium and lead to plaque buildup. A study published in the journal *Atherosclerosis* reinforcess the fact that healthy HDL levels can protect the endothelium and prevent against LDL oxidation. Furthermore, when levels of triglycerides, a type of fat present in the blood, are high, they can bind with LDL cholesterol, enter the vessel wall, and form plaque more aggressively and efficiently than LDL alone.

High insulin and high blood glucose (sugar) also contribute to endothelial dysfunction and accelerate the development of atherosclerosis (hardening of the arteries). High glucose levels also prompt the pancreas to produce more insulin, so it's a vicious cycle that can accelerate CVD.

Finally, hypertension, or high blood pressure, increases the amount of force as blood flows across the endothelium. The higher your blood pressure, the more pressure is exerted on the vessel walls and endothelial cells, causing micro-tears in the endothelium, which compromise its integrity. Consistently high pressure can damage the endothelial cells and lead to endothelial dysfunction and, as a result, CVD. (For more on blood pressure, see "Measuring Your Progress," page 90.)

What's particularly harmful about the five "highs" is that once the process of damage begins, additional damage occurs. Each of the dysfunctional states lead to endothelial dysfunction, but a dysfunctional endothelium feeds these issues, too. Dysfunction leads to more dysfunction.

Stress

Stress isn't always a bad thing. "Good" stress, known as eustress, is positive pressure that motivates a person to excel or succeed. It's what encourages an employee to work harder, an athlete to train longer, and a physician to push through the long hours of medical school. Exercise also puts positive pressure, or stress, on the body that contributes to wellness. But there is a flip side known as distress, which can cause a lot of harm to the body.

Distress is the natural stress reaction of the "fight or flight mechanism" and can either be good or bad. Think of the well-known "bear in the woods" example: You're walking through the forest, minding your own business. Suddenly, a large bear appears in your path. It stands up on its hind legs, its body extended, ready to eat you whole. What do you do? You must either run away (flight) or stand your ground and try to scare it away (fight). Instead of wasting time weighing the options, good distress causes the body to instantly respond to danger.

Distress can also give you "super powers." It provides the body with a rush of adrenaline that helps a person run faster or have incredible strength. Have you ever heard of a person lifting a car off the ground to save someone underneath? That's adrenaline at work, and it's good distress because, in this case, it can save a person's life.

The problem today is that people are under distress for long periods of time. Distress is meant to be a momentary thing, something that lasts for short bursts, only present during a crisis situation. But too much distress over a long period of time—known as chronic stress— can have terrible effects. Chronic stress causes the body to continually release the stress hormone cortisol into the blood stream. While the body needs cortisol, constant excessive amounts can cause a host of issues, including insomnia, higher insulin levels, and excess fat storage.

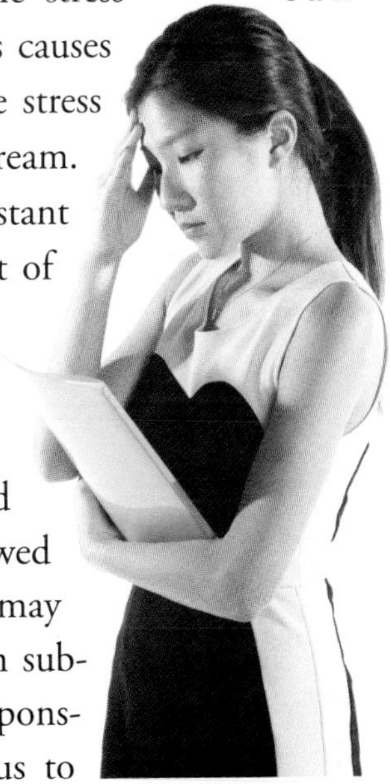

An in-depth study conducted by the University of Helsinki showed that "both chronic and acute stress may exert an effect on atherosclerosis in subjects with impaired endothelial responses." In short, good stress moves us to action. When bad stress—either short (acute) or, especially, chronic—stays bottled up inside with no physical release, it damages the endothelium. And, as you've learned, endothelial dysfunction is the first step toward CVD.

Sleep

Sleep is one of the most important activities you can do because it heals and restores your body. When you don't get enough sleep, it can be detrimental to the health of your endothelium. Nighttime is when your endothelium—the workhorse of the cardiovascular system—gets to take a break and rest.

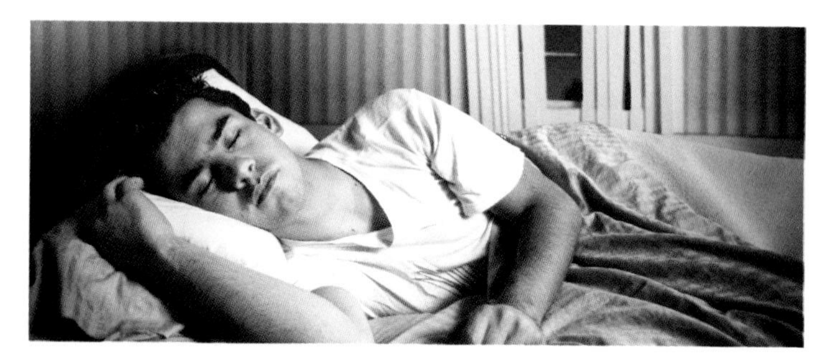

Inadequate sleep can result in high blood pressure and elevated blood sugar levels—two of the five "highs." It also impacts hormone levels and negatively affects the secretory functions of the endothelium, including NO production. Obstructive sleep apnea, a condition that can cause high blood pressure, is associated with endothelial dysfunction. Researchers have also found that people who are sleep-deprived eat an average of 221 more calories a day—and we're willing to bet those aren't nutrient-dense calories.

Smoking

Smoking has an immediate effect on the endothelium through increased free radical damage that instantly impairs endothelial dysfunction. (For more on free radical damage, see page 48.) Many people know nicotine in tobacco is a vasoconstrictor, meaning it causes the blood vessels to narrow, but there's more to it. When a person smokes tobacco, you may notice his face flush. That's because the chemicals are causing immediate vasodilation, or expansion of the blood vessels. Sounds good, right? Well, there's also an instant rebound of the blood vessels know as vasoconstriction. That expansion and constriction caused by nicotine and other chemicals in tobacco is what causes the physical stress and resulting damage to the endothelium.

Here's the bottom line: smoking leads to endothelial dysfunction. Good nutrition, targeted supplementation, regular exercise, and other positive changes won't overcome the detrimental effects of smoking. It's bad for the whole body, but it's especially damaging to the endothelium and entire cardiovascular system.

Age

Even the best diet and exercise regimen can't stop aging. It can slow the impact, but it can't halt the process altogether. Just like your skin forms wrinkles or your knees start aching, endothelial function also declines with age.

Here's what happens: As endothelial cells age, they aren't able to regenerate or self-heal as easily as they could in younger years. The endothelium's protective functions weaken and leaks form, opening up the walls of the ar-

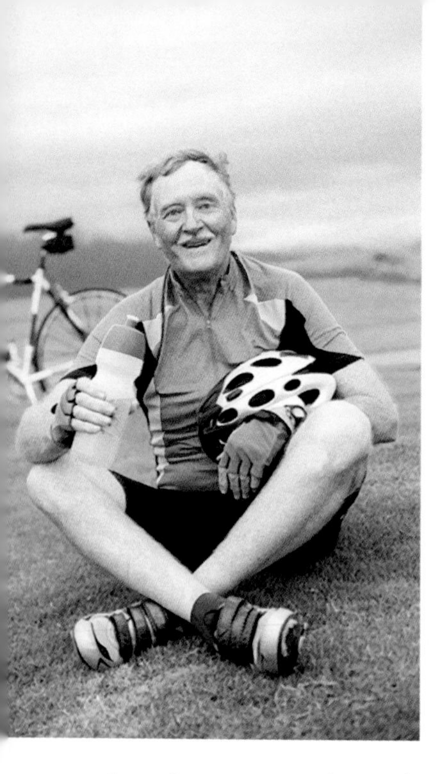

teries to damage. Some of the signaling functions, including NO production, decrease; since signals from the endothelium are necessary to the function of the arteries, the arteries are unable to react as they should. When the smooth muscles within the arterial wall sense this decline, it reacts by sending smooth muscle cells to the surface of the endothelium. And what does that cause? Atherosclerosis, or hardening of the arteries, one of the key markers for heart disease.

There are multiple factors that cause endothelial dysfunction. Thankfully, all but one of them are preventable. You can't stop aging, but you can avoid the damaging outcomes by staying active, eating a healthy diet, maintaining your weight, avoiding the five "highs," lowering stress levels, getting plenty of sleep, and not smoking. In Section 3, we'll explore exactly what a healthy lifestyle looks like, as well as detail supplemental nutrients that can enhance endothelial function.

Younger and Younger

A few decades ago, people died of heart disease all the time, and CVD was a leading cause of death, just like it is now. But, back then, it was a disease of the aged; people rarely died from heart disease until they were well into their golden years. Signs of heart disease tended to show up later in life, when people were in their sixties, seventies, or later. But there is a marked difference today: CVD-related deaths are not uncommon in people in their fifties, or even forties. Cardiovascular dysfunction is no longer typical only in older adults—it's an epidemic impacting people of almost any age, beginning in childhood. Here are some startling facts:

- Endothelial dysfunction can begin as early as the first decade of life. That means heart disease can start before a child turns ten years old!

- In the past thirty years, childhood obesity has tripled. A 2010 CDC study showed that more than one-third of the children surveyed were overweight or obese.

- Kids who show signs of endothelial dysfunction may end up developing heart disease in their twenties or thirties instead of their sixties or seventies.

What's causing the early arrival of cardiovascular dysfunction? In past generations, kids were more active; they spent their days running around outside with friends instead of inside playing video games or surfing the Internet. Fast food, sodas, and other unhealthy options weren't read-

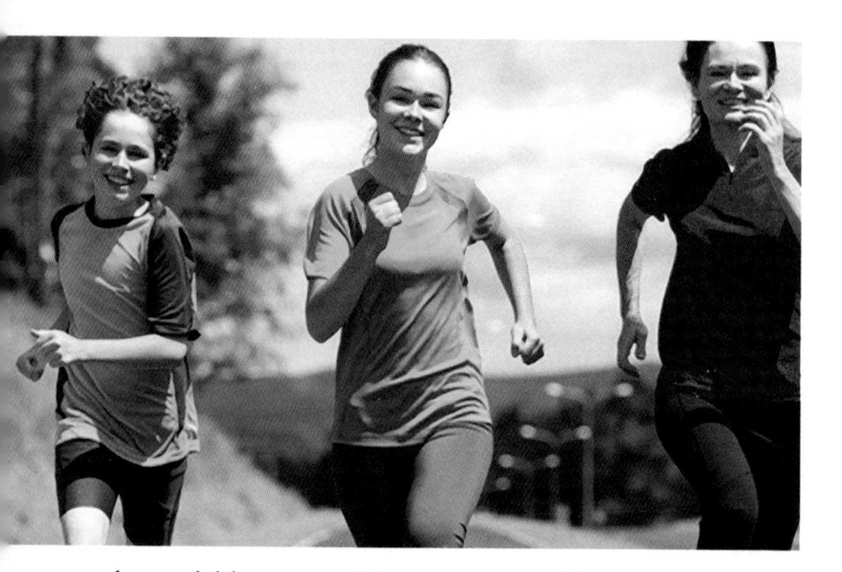

ily available—or widely consumed—like they are today. Modern lifestyle and diet are causing kids to get fatter and fatter and their endothelium to become more and more dysfunctional. Children are also now being diagnosed with Type 2 diabetes, a condition that used to be referred to as "adult onset." But it's no longer just an adult's disease. A kid who's inactive and eats a standard American diet may end up with Type 2 diabetes before they're done with their teenage years.

The age at which endothelium dysfunction begins is the starting point for heart disease. It's when you click the button on the CVD stopwatch; the sooner endothelial dysfunction starts, the sooner heart disease will strike.

On a Continuum: The 3D Effect and Endothelial Dysfunction

We wrote *Health Is Wealth* to help redefine and reapproach disease from a completely different point of view and offer strategies for living a vital, full life. As we reviewed scientific studies for the book, we noticed that there were volumes of published clinical research that identified nutrient deficiency and its negative impact on health. We started to dig deeper, searching for connections that would help us share a new approach to health and wellness—a preventive focus. We found two things:

1. Multiple peer-reviewed scientific studies clearly indicate that nutritional deficiency is the base cause of what conventional medicine diagnoses as disease.

2. Modern lifestyle creates nutrient depletion, to the extent that even a relatively healthy diet doesn't contain enough nutrients to keep the body functioning optimally.

Applying Dr. Myers's naturopathic approach helped us come up with the term "Nutrient Deficiency Syndrome" (NDS) to describe the *real* cause of dysfunction in the body. It works like this: Modern lifestyle puts an incredible amount of stress on the body, which increases nutritional needs. From job layoffs to constant travel to family problems, ours is a culture constantly under pressure. Add to that the availability of processed, high-fat foods, inactivity, poor sleep habits, excess weight, and a myriad of other issues. Since modern diet usually compounds the problem, our poor bodies are suffering from severe nutrient depletion. That's what NDS describes.

You may not be showing any obvious signs of nutritional deficiency. But if you're not getting key nutrients, your body is functioning suboptimally. You might feel tired, groggy, fatigued, or just not "well." You might be overweight. You might have trouble sleeping or become tired partway through the day. These are all the signs of NDS. The hard part about these early symptoms is they're hard to measure and quantify.

Let's look at the concept of NDS another way. Say you go visit the doctor for a checkup. You're diagnosed with high cholesterol and given a prescription statin drug to help lower your cholesterol levels. A diagnosis of high cholesterol doesn't specifically describe the dysfunction that's being driven by nutrient deficiency, and taking a statin drug isn't dealing with the real problem, which is poor diet and lifestyle choices. Not only that, but statins can decrease CoQ10 in the body, a critical coenzyme involved in energy production. So, taking a statin causes you to become more and more deficient in CoQ10, leading to additional "symptoms of disease." Those symptoms are really just your body's way of telling you that it's missing some key nutrients.

We combined our expertise with the research we reviewed to describe what we call the 3D Effect: **depletion** leads to **deficiency**, which ultimately leads to **dysfunction**, or what conventional medicine would diagnose as "disease." It's a devastating continuum that takes years, often decades, to come into full effect. We describe the 3D Effect and

NDS in depth in *Health Is Wealth* in relation to total body wellness. Here, we look at it in terms of the cardiovascular system:

1. **Depletion** is the initial drop of one or more essential nutrients the endothelium needs to function optimally. This can be caused by poor lifestyle choices that involve diet, sleep, and movement, among others. These stress the endothelium physiologically, and these stressors will deplete the functional nutrients at an even quicker pace. As the endothelium becomes depleted of nutrition, we begin to see changes in its functionality, including a decreased capacity for production of NO. This can lead to an impaired response of the endothelium in its control of vasodilation and will eventually lead to increased blood pressure. 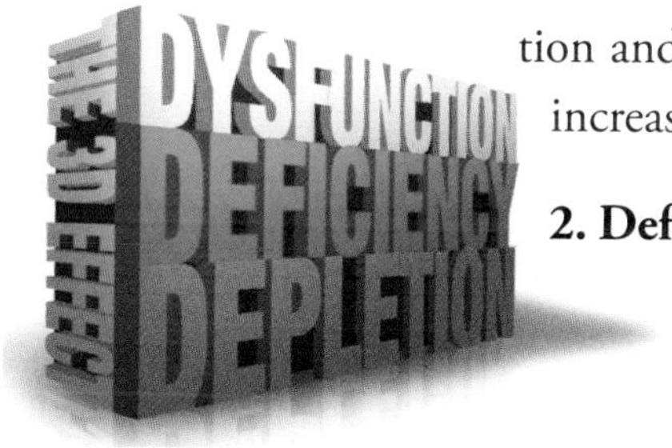
2. **Deficiency** occurs when the endothelium has been deprived of one or more essential nutrients over a long period of time, causing the individual endothelial cells to weaken or die, creating holes and gaps. Deficiency makes the endothelium's natural regeneration process, which is running on empty, more difficult or even impossible. The holes and gaps that form in the endothelium make it susceptible to leakage of cholesterol, fats, and other cellular waste. Plaque may begin to build up in the arterial wall, causing the arteries to start the hardening process that leads to athero-

sclerosis. As the endothelium becomes deficient in nutrition, elevated blood pressure, due to chronic insufficiency of NO, is almost always present. In addition, as deficiency extends to involve other nutrients critical to endothelial function, we see increased damage from free radical oxidation leading to further degradation of function.

3. **Dysfunction** begins when enough damage has been done to the endothelial cells to impair function and then manifest as symptoms. This is a long process and can take decades to reach the dysfunction stage. With chronic, multiple nutritional deficiencies, the endothelium can no longer protect itself or the cardiovascular system, and dysfunction will progress into a heart attack, stroke, or some other catastrophic event.

It's important to understand that obesity is the starting point of NDS in CVD. Remember, excess fat isn't just unattractive—those excess fat (lipid) cells release harmful chemicals and hormones into the body. Obesity puts the body in a constant state of inflammation and can lead to metabolic syndrome, then Type 2 diabetes, and eventually to CVD. Obesity is the starting point of almost all CVD (and disease in general, for that matter). By the time a person becomes obese, he or she is already in a state of nutritional depletion or deficiency, heading toward dysfunction.

Modern Lifestyle Isn't Changing

Let's just say you eat a perfect diet, which should provide all of the nutrients you need. When you layer in the stress typical of our world today, the body's need for nutrients increases, because stress is a process that causes additional damage and creates greater nutritional needs. The bottom line? Modern lifestyle depletes the body, which can eventually progress to a deficiency state…and, in the end, lead to dysfunction.

The fact is that our world isn't changing. Chronic stress isn't going away any time soon, and we don't foresee fast food restaurants closing shop. More and more ways to avoid physical movement crop up all the time. You might not be able to avoid depleting your endothelium. But you *can* change deficiency by making better choices and supplementing with Power Nutrients for endothelial health, which we'll detail in Section 3.

One thing our review of published research shows is that nutrients work together. Double-blind, peer-reviewed studies often try to isolate nutrients to understand their role in the body. But that's a very limited way of looking at the body because nutrients work as a team, keeping the body healthy together. It's the same with deficiency of the endothelium. Once you have a core group of nutritional deficiencies impacting the endothelial cells, it actually breeds additional deficiencies in the cardiovascular system because the endothelium is trying to compensate for the nutrients it's lacking. It's a compensatory effect in which the initial deficiencies breed more deficiencies within the body.

Case Study: Oscar and the Dysfunctional Endothelium

You met our study subject, Kim, in Section 1 (see page 39). As you might recall, Kim has a healthy endothelium because she makes great choices most of the time and supplements with Power Nutrients to fill the nutritional gaps that occur. Now, meet Oscar.

Oscar is a fifty-six-year-old male who leads a typical American lifestyle: minimal movement and excess sitting; a diet of high-fat, processed foods and very little fresh produce; continual stress at work and home; and just five-and-a-half to six hours of sleep most nights. As you might have guessed, Oscar also has a weight problem; he's carrying an extra fifty pounds of fat. His most recent visit to the doctor revealed that the metabolic syndrome and prediabetes he's been dealing with for years has now progressed to Type 2 diabetes. His blood pressure is high and triglyceride levels are worrisome. Basically, he's sick and getting sicker.

Let's look at Oscar's daily routine. To save time, he skips breakfast. After arriving at work, he drinks the first of several cups of coffee with ample milk and sugar. He picks up lunch at a fast food restaurant, hurries back to work, and eats his deep fried chicken sandwich (with extra mayo and cheese), fries, and 24-ounce soft drink while catching up on e-mails. This high-fat, low-nutrient lunch puts pressure on his already dysfunctional endothelium. Since the cells are damaged and the body's already in a state of chronic inflammation, it just causes more damage to the endothelium, leaving the vessel walls even more compromised. Now, since holes are starting to form in the endothelium, cholesterol and fats enter the vessel wall, causing the endothelium to call for help in the form of white blood cells. A number of chemical processes cause those white blood cells to start the process of turning into plaque. And this process happens each and every time Oscar eats an unhealthy meal.

During his workday, Oscar only stands four times: twice to use the bathroom, once to ask a subordinate a question, and once more to help himself to the doughnuts he spotted in the break room. He reasons that if there are still some doughnuts left before he leaves for the day, he'll have another. In total, he's away from his desk for eighteen minutes out of the four hours he works after lunch. Because of his sedentary day, Oscar's endothelial cells aren't stimulated to produce NO. His NO levels are already low because of the damage from his diet, stress, sleep, and other issues. And since NO signals the blood vessels to dilate, lack of the critical molecule contributes to high blood pressure, among other issues.

After work, Oscar drives the thirty-minute commute home during rush hour. Driving stresses him out. As he honks at one driver and yells at another, he feels his chest tighten and breath quicken. His body releases cortisol as a response to deal with the stressor. But the problem is that this "fight or flight" response happens throughout much of his day, with no relief from his internal distress. High cortisol levels contribute to atherosclerosis, or hardening of the arteries. Since this has been going on for over a decade, Oscar's arteries are far along the atherosclerotic process.

On the outside, Oscar looks unhealthy. On the inside, he looks unhealthy, too. His blood vessels are bumpy with plaque buildup and his arteries are hardening. His endothelium has pockets of dead and damaged cells, so the endothelial cells aren't able to produce the hormones, chemicals, and molecules necessary to regulate blood flow. Because his endothelium is dysfunctional, NO levels are low, and his vessels aren't able to dilate properly. His blood is thick and sticky. There is a lot of pressure on his vessel walls as the heart works extra hard to pump his thick blood through inflexible vessels. Oscar is destined for a heart attack or stroke...and it'll happen sooner rather than later.

Every day, Oscar takes one more step on the road to CVD. His body is trying everything it can to heal the damage he's doing, but it can't overcome constant negative input. He needs to change his habits now. What's amazing about the human body is that, even with all of the damage he's caused, it's not too late for Oscar to completely reverse endothelial dysfunction and restore the health of his endothelial cells. And it's not too late for you, either.

The Great News: Reversing Endothelial Dysfunction

There's some amazing news we haven't discussed in depth yet: endothelial dysfunction is **reversible**.

Remember the 3D Effect, the continuum from depletion to dysfunction? It's not a one-way continuum. Your body has incredible, innate healing mechanisms that can reverse almost any condition. But it needs the right input to have the chance to restore function.

> There's some amazing news we haven't discussed in depth yet: endothelial dysfunction is **reversible**.

Think about it this way: When you are injured externally—a cut, bruise, or scrape, for example—your body self-heals. There may be a small mark left over in the form of a scar, but you're usually otherwise fine, right? It's the same with your endothelium. The difference is that, for your endothelium to be able to restore balance, it absolutely must have key nutrients, and you need to stop damaging the endothelial cells.

It's a continuum, but it's a reversible, two-way continuum. If you're progressing toward dysfunction, you can turn around and head in the other direction toward function and wellness. Even if you have full-blown heart disease, you can literally repair and rebuild your cardiovascular system. You may have to take some extreme actions to return to health, but, in most cases, it's 100 percent possible. It is *never* too late.

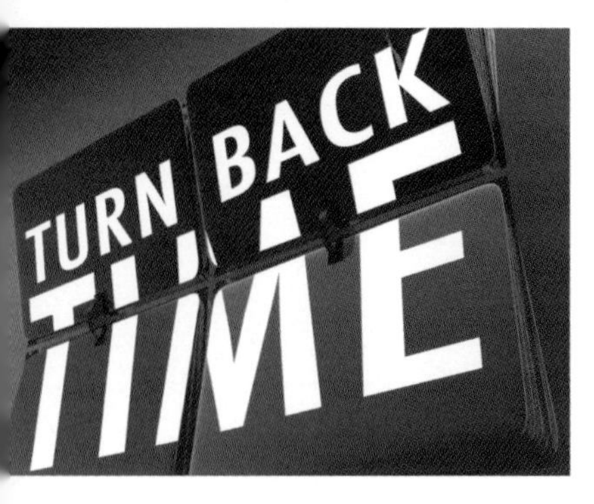

We're going to be straightforward with you: getting healthy isn't easy. But if you make the radical changes needed to reverse endothelial dysfunction, you will begin to see positive changes to your cardiovascular system—even if you're currently on multiple medications or facing surgery. It doesn't matter where you are in a disease process with regards to heart disease. There's always hope.

Reframing the Approach

We've already redefined disease as the manifestation of symptoms that result from a long progression toward dysfunction. Now, we'd like to reiterate that the *approach* toward wellness will be totally different than what the conventional medical system suggests.

Consider the last time you went to the doctor with an earache, sinus infection, or other issue. You probably got a prescription. When you took that prescription, you likely expected to wake up the next day feeling at least a little better.

When it comes to CVD, people often take a similar approach. Take a pill, get better, right? Wrong. You might feel better in the short term, but your cardiovascular system won't be functioning at its peak. Long-term prescription drugs have their own troublesome side effects, and they're not fixing the problem. Cardiovascular medications are just

Band-Aids for dysfunction of the cardiovascular system, dysfunction that began with the tiny endothelial cells that line those one hundred thousand miles of blood vessels in your body.

Approaching endothelial dysfunction from a holistic perspective takes a more proactive approach. Research shows that the only way to repair the endothelium is to make positive changes—eat healthier, move more, maintain a healthy weight, get more sleep, and reduce stress. But many people struggle with consistency and patience. It takes consistent, concerted lifestyle changes over a long period of time to reverse the devastating effects of endothelial dysfunction. And it takes patience, because the process is slow, and there aren't many noticeable milestones by which to measure progress.

If you're a parent, do you remember holding your newborn baby in your arms? As your baby grew, it was as though you blinked, and all of a sudden your tiny newborn was three, six, nine, and then twelve months old. You probably weren't aware of the day-to-day changes and developments. Sure, you noticed major milestones like baby's first laugh or step, but were you able to perceive the incremental progression each and every day—her length, weight, eye tracking, or how fluidly she moved her hands to grasp an object? Looking back on the photos or videos of your baby's first year, though, there were huge leaps and bounds. Daily advancements eventually equaled major growth and development. You weren't able to notice those small changes, the gradual advancements she made every day, because they were too subtle to notice.

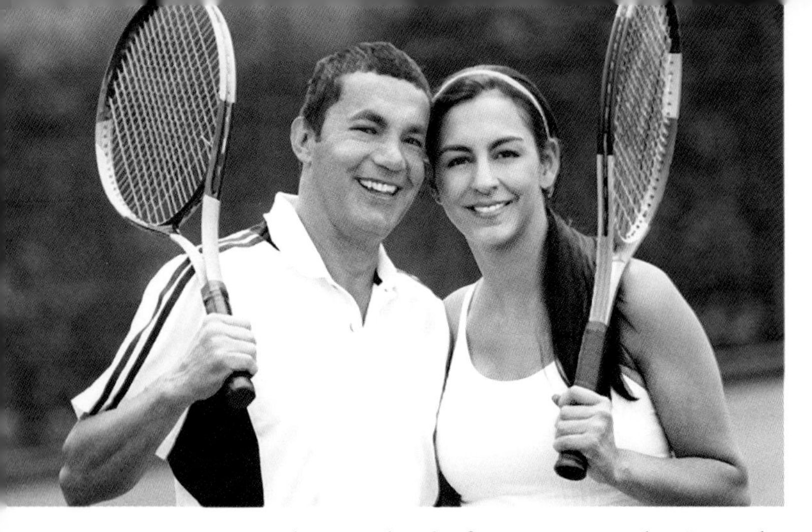

Reversing cardiovascular dysfunction is similar. It can be hard to see the results of the good decisions you make each and every day. It's when you've been making those choices for three, six, nine, or twelve months, and continue them throughout your entire life, that you begin to notice the incredible progress you've made. That transitional period can be discouraging at times, because the "quick fix" and immediate response we're used to as a society aren't part of a natural, holistic approach.

We like to describe prescription drugs as a sledgehammer and lifestyle changes as a finishing hammer. The sledgehammer works faster, but it's imprecise and can cause more damage. A finishing hammer takes a lot longer to do the job, but it's more exact and careful. The finishing hammer approach to cardiovascular wellness slowly, carefully, and effectively restores health. It's progressive improvement.

If you have life-threatening heart disease, or any other serious disease, for that matter, we're not telling you to stop taking your prescription. By all means, take the prescription to stay alive. But, in the meantime, start a proactive transformation, one that will leave you empowered, energized, and even add years to your life. Be sure to talk to a physician trained in holistic medicine to help create a wellness plan tailored to your specific circumstance.

Change Takes Time

People often ask us how long it will take to see a difference in their cardiovascular health once they start making positive lifestyle changes. That's a hard question to answer because every body is different. In general, it takes at least three months of a consistently healthy lifestyle to begin to see the reversal of endothelial dysfunction. Really, that's a minimum, but it is a point when you should start noticing the benefits of your hard work.

There are some exceptions to this. Vitamin C, for example, can improve endothelial function almost immediately. A study in the American Heart Association's journal *Circulation* showed that vitamin C supplements result in "increased availability of nitric oxide." Since NO is the signaling molecule that is involved in vasodilation (widening of blood vessels), taking vitamin C can have a near-instant impact on blood flow. But while vitamin C is a great support to endothelial function on an immediate basis, restoration of function and lasting change take time.

It takes years to damage your endothelium and undo the natural state of health and vitality in your cardiovascular system. It will take several months of consistent, concerted efforts to start restoring endothelial health.

While it may seem like a long time, it's actually remarkable how quickly the body repairs itself. Let's say you've been unhealthy for twenty years. Fast food, no exercise, smoking, you name it. Then, one day, you decide you're ready to get healthy. Within minutes of stopping smoking, the endothelium begins to repair itself. The first balanced meal you eat delivers key nutrients to your cardiovascular system and starts the process toward wellness. The first walk or jog you take gets your blood pumping, which stimulates your endothelial cells and encourages the production of NO.

While you may not start to feel or see the impacts of those good choices for many months, your body begins the process right away. The same is true of nutritional supplementation; the results on a cellular level take effect immediately, but it takes a while for the overall condition of the endothelium to be repaired. Even if it takes a year or two to get your body to function optimally, that's a pretty short time frame, considering the years or decades of damage. And it's not just your endothelium that starts repairing itself; your entire body begins restoring function, as well. It's incredible.

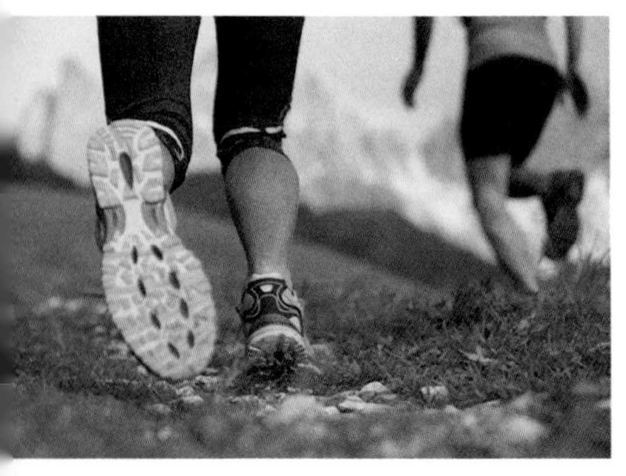

With that very first step you take toward getting healthy, you're *already* on your way to reversing endothelial dysfunction. In Section 3, we'll explain what a healthy lifestyle looks like, as well as detail 10 Power Nutrients that can help restore the health of the endothelium—and prevent or reverse heart disease.

The moment you start making good lifestyle choices, the body begins to heal itself. It doesn't matter how unhealthy you are today. If you replace bad habits with good ones tomorrow, you start on the path toward health.

Section 3

Strategies for a Healthy Endothelium

Imagine yourself ten, twenty, even thirty or more years from now. How do you look and feel in your older age? As a naturopathic physician, Dr. Myers has treated patients ranging from sick, immobile sixty-year-olds to vital, active ninety-year-olds. The difference isn't usually genetics. In most cases, the reason some people *live* until they die—as opposed to just getting through life one day at a time—is because they make consistently great choices over many, many years.

Age is just a number. You can't change your biological age, but you can improve how your body responds to age. Because most cells in the body regenerate, it's possible to maintain the youth and functionality of your cells until you're very old. Of course, there are certain cells and organs of the body that can't be renewed; brain cortical neurons have a fixed number of cells from birth that naturally decline with aging, for example. But, through a holistic approach to wellness, you could be healthy and vital well into your eighties and nineties. And since your cardiovascular

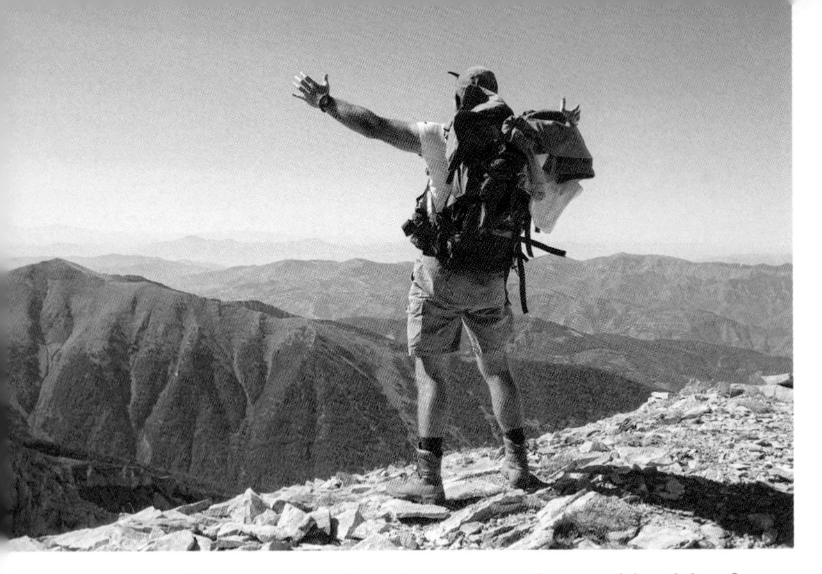

system has a tremendous impact on the total health of your body, we recommend that the starting place for vitality is the endothelium.

Now, we know that all of this critical information about your endothelium is useless without providing real, doable steps that you can follow to restore endothelial health and prevent or reverse cardiovascular disease (CVD). Understanding reversibility and restoration is great, but the *how* is the most important element.

In the next pages, we'll present a proven approach to reversing endothelial dysfunction. It begins with changing the way you think, move, eat, and sleep. Our regimen doesn't involve a fad diet or sixty-day workout regimen. It's not something you can do for a few months and then quit. It's a lifetime commitment, a shift in mind-set. It's a proactive approach, not a reactive one. You have the power to shape your future and live a life of vitality. You can add years to your life and improve the quality of each and every moment from here on out.

We'd like to make an important point: positive choices don't completely counteract harmful ones. Smoking, drinking alcohol (with the exception of red wine in moderation), and exposure to other toxic substances can easily undo all of the hard work you're putting into getting healthy. We know it can be difficult to quit. But quitting smoking and use of other tobacco products, as well as limiting alcohol consumption, can be among the most important health decisions you will make, period. Be sure to talk to your physician for advice and support.

It's All About Lifestyle

Recall the image you formed in the previous section of yourself in your older age. Now, envision the way your future could look: You're eighty years old and feel great. On a typical Saturday, you go to brunch and take a morning hike, play piano at the community center, and go dancing in the early evening. At the end of your long, active day, you retire to bed and sleep soundly through the night. The best part is that you've been living healthy, vital, and alive for decades.

Could this be possible for you? Absolutely.

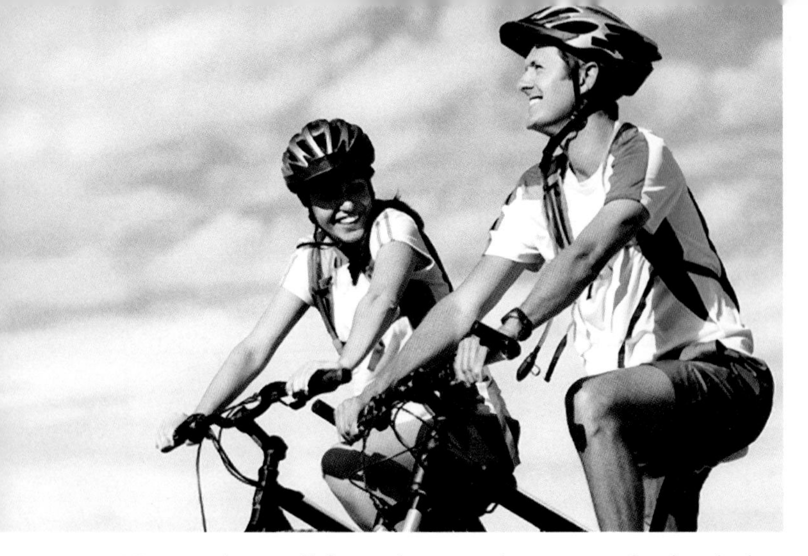

You might recall from the introduction to this book that health is freedom. Being healthy allows you to live the life you want well into your old age. Almost anyone can do so. The first step is adopting a healthy lifestyle; the second step is supplementing with critical nutrients. We'll look at the lifestyle piece first.

Living a healthy lifestyle isn't as complicated as it might seem. It's pretty simple, really: eat a balanced, nutritious diet that includes the 10 Power Nutrients for endothelial health and plenty of water; get regular exercise and lots of daily movement; lower your stress levels; and get at least eight hours of sleep per night. The hard part comes in when you have to stick with your new commitment and see it through. Some people can easily adjust; others will wait until their first heart attack to finally change. Which will you be?

Eating for a Healthy Endothelium

Wholesome food is the basis of a healthy endothelium, and we recommend what is known as the Mediterranean diet to support endothelial health. Rich in foods frequently found in the countries along the Mediterranean Sea, the diet includes most of the healthy staples: fresh fruits and vegetables, protein, whole grains, and fish. But it also incorporates some unique additions like olive oil and red wine.

According to the Mayo Clinic, research has shown that adhering to the Mediterranean diet reduces the risk of heart disease. An analysis of over 1.5 million healthy adults showed that eating the Mediterranean diet was not only associated with reduced incidence of heart disease but also of cancer, Parkinson's, and Alzheimer's. Separate research also found that the "Mediterranean diet reduces endothelial damage and improves the regenerative capacity of the endothelium." Numerous other scientific studies have shown the incredible power of the Mediterranean diet on cardiovascular health as well.

Plant-based foods like fruits, vegetables, whole grains, olive oil, nuts, beans, seeds, legumes, and herbs and spices make up the biggest portion of the heart-healthy Mediterranean diet. Healthy fats like olive oil are used instead of saturated fats like butter. (Keep in mind that olive oil is a medium-temperature oil; cooking it at a high temperature will cause it to lose some of its healthful qualities.) Herbs and spices replace salt for adding flavor to dishes.

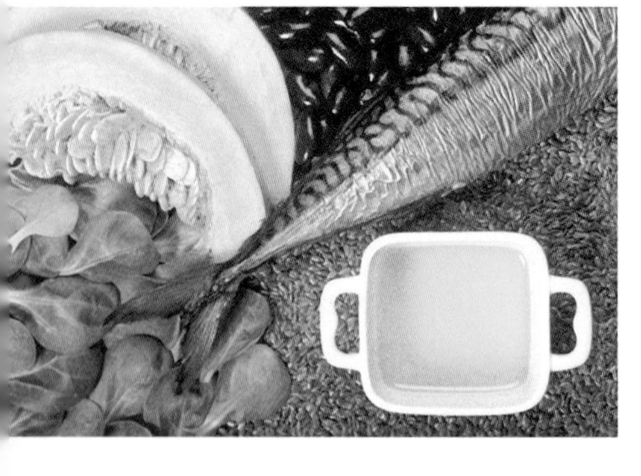

Red meat should be limited to no more than a few times a month. Fish and poultry should make up most of the meat intake and be eaten at least twice per week. Red wine can be added, if desired, for its antioxidant benefits.

The Mediterranean diet is great for your endothelium. By limiting foods rich in Omega-6, which are essential and healthy but can cause inflammation when consumed in excess, the diet supports a balanced intake of Omega-6s and Omega-3s. It places emphasis on whole foods like vegetables and fruits, which provide your endothelium with the nutrients it needs to function at its peak. The diet limits the foods that put stress on the endothelium: high-fat foods, salt, processed foods, and refined sugar. With supplementation, the benefits of Mediterranean eating multiply.

Other foods to add to your endothelium-boosting diet include green tea, garlic, cocoa, pomegranates, and beets. Since oxidative stress is a major contributor to endothelial dysfunction, green tea's powerful antioxidant qualities help neutralize free radical damage and restore the endothelium. A study published in the *European Journal of Cardiovascular Prevention and Rehabilitation* found that green tea has an "acute beneficial effect on the endothelium" in healthy individuals. Other studies have found that green tea can even help heal the endothelium from the effects of smoking. It's astounding that a tiny tea leaf can do so much good for the cardiovascular system.

Garlic has been shown to reduce inflammation and potentially reverse atherosclerosis (hardening of the arteries). Research published in the *American Journal of Clinical Nutrition* even showed that dark chocolate and liquid cocoa improved endothelial function and lowered blood pressure in overweight adults. Of course, moderation is key when it comes to sweets like dark chocolate and cocoa, but they are incredibly powerful when consumed in limited amounts. Pomegranate has been shown to increase nitric oxie (NO), which supports the function of the endothelial cells. And finally, beets are endothelium-boosting miracles. A study in the American Heart Association's journal *Hypertension* showed that beetroot juice lowers blood pressure and prevents endothelial dysfunction, as well as offers a natural, cost-effective option for treating CVD. We'll look at some of these in greater depth when we discuss the 10 Power Nutrients for endothelial health.

For more information on the Mediterranean diet, we recommend the nonprofit organization Oldways (oldwayspt.org), which offers free information and recipes for people wanting to follow the Mediterranean diet. Our website, HealthIsWealth.net, is also a great resource for healthy eating and living.

Get Moving for Endothelial Health

Without good nutrition, your endothelium can't function optimally; it's just not possible. As you work on implementing or continuing an endothelium-healthy diet,

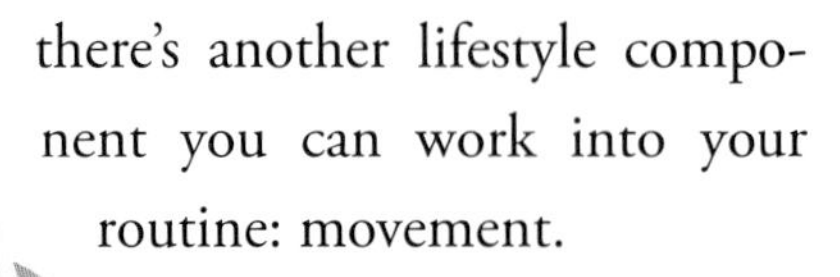

there's another lifestyle component you can work into your routine: movement.

Our bodies are made to move. Physical activity has all sorts of positive effects on the body. It improves symptoms of mood disorders like depression, helps prevent bone loss (osteoporosis), balances and supports healthy blood sugar levels, improves sleep, and helps in weight loss and maintenance, among other benefits. But most important to our discussion is the remarkable effect physical activity has on the endothelium.

Movement of any kind—walking, running, snowshoeing, ballroom dancing—increases blood flow within the arteries. This increased blood flow is known as "shear stress." As the blood moves across the endothelium (which lines the interior of the artery), it stimulates the individual cells, causing an increase in NO production. And, as we've learned, NO is the most important molecule in the entire cardiovascular system. The more NO your body produces, the healthier your heart will be.

Lifelong athletes increase NO each and every day. As they engage in their sports of choice, movement consistently stimulates their endothelial cells to produce additional NO. Have you ever noticed that athletes tend to look younger than they are? That's due, in part, to NO's role as an antioxidant. If you could take an internal photo of an athlete's body, he or she would look young on the inside, too. In most cases, athletes' arteries are smooth and flexible, their blood pressure is within normal range, and the endothelium is functioning optimally, creating and regulating all of the chemicals, hormones, and molecules needed to keep the arteries plaque-free. And the benefits of continual movement don't stop there. Regular movement trains your endothelial cells to produce more NO *consistently*, not just when you're exercising. Your baseline NO production improves.

Getting the CDC's recommended 150 minutes of exercise is excellent, but it's even better to get more. We recommend a minimum of thirty minutes of physical activity a day, five or six days a week. And we'll add to that: you should move whenever, wherever, and however you can. A study in the *British Medical Journal* showed that just by sitting less, you can increase your life expectancy by up to two years or more!

Do you work in an office? Get a "standing desk," take walking breaks throughout the day, pace your office while on the phone, or find other ways to work movement into your otherwise sedentary workday. Just standing or pacing during phone calls and using a tall filing cabinet as a desktop while you take notes can burn an extra 100 to 130 calories per day. When you go to the grocery store, park far away from the door; you'll do your heart a favor by adding an extra 150 or so steps from the car to the entryway. Go on a walk with your family each evening after dinner. Keep the television off on the weekends and go for a family bike ride instead. Take the stairs instead of the elevator. Each of these small actions adds up to a healthier endothelium.

Measuring Your Progress

There is currently no easy way to diagnose endothelial dysfunction. Perhaps the future will bring a quick in-office test to assess endothelial health. But since one doesn't yet exist, you'll have to use other methods for assessing how your endothelial cells are functioning. A simple, free, and fast way to get an idea of the health of your endothelium is through a blood pressure test.

When blood pressure is within normal range, it's a good indicator of endothelial health. Why? Vasodilation. "Vaso" means vessel; "dilate" means open. So, vasodilation is when the vessels widen. This was covered in Section 1, but we'd like to take a moment to recap.

Arteries, veins, and capillaries are all forms of blood vessels that perform different functions in the body. In this case, we're looking at the arteries, since they have the smooth muscle that allows expansion or contraction of the vessel to alter blood flow in response to pressure on the arterial wall. When the endothelium is healthy, it responds instantly to this pressure, as well as to demands from the tissues in the body, and produces more NO, which causes vasodilation. When arteries widen, blood flows more easily through the cardiovascular system, nourishing the heart and other critical organs.

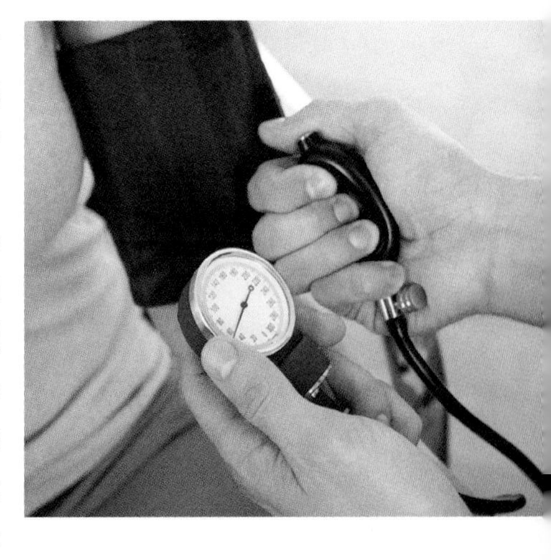

Blood pressure is the pressure the blood exerts on the blood vessel walls as it flows through the body. This pressure is at its highest during systole (heart contraction), just before the blood leaves the heart (in the aorta), and lowest when the heart is relaxed during diastole (heart dilation) and is preparing to beat again, just before blood reenters the heart (through the venae cavae). The American Heart Association recommends that blood pressure levels should be less than 120/80. The higher number (systolic) is the maximum pressure that the blood exerts. The lowest number (diastolic) is the minimum pressure the blood exerts. The numbers are measured in "millimeters of mercury," or mm Hg. Blood pressure is affected by many things including diet, exercise levels, fitness levels, cholesterol levels, smoking, and stress, just to name a few.

In order to assess the health of your endothelium, we recommend taking a blood pressure test. Your doctor can do this for you, you can get it done for free at a local pharmacy, or you can purchase a relatively inexpensive at-home blood pressure monitor. If your endothelium is healthy, your blood pressure will be within normal range. Be sure you aren't stressed and haven't just heavily exerted yourself.

You can access a guide to understanding what "normal range" means for your specific body and medical condition at the American Heart Association's website, heart.org (search for "Understanding Blood Pressure Readings").

After you take your initial test, check your blood pressure once a week and record the number; try to test around the same time and under the same conditions each week. In your log, note the date and time, along with your blood pressure, heart rate, and stress level from zero to ten, with zero being completely relaxed and ten being stressed to the max. As your endothelium becomes healthier, you will see your blood pressure readings drop and other heart function tests improve. As your endothelial function improves and your heart get stronger, your heart rate may also drop slightly. These are all great indications of the health of your endothelium.

Here's a fun activity: you can convert the millimeters of mercury (mm Hg) to pounds of pressure per square inch (psi) to get a good idea of the actual pressure your blood is putting on your vessel walls. Here's the equation:

mm Hg x 0.0193367747 = psi

So, for example, blood pressure within normal range would be:

120 mm Hg x 0.0193367747 = 2.3 psi
(systolic; approximate maximum pressure)

80 mm Hg x 0.0193367747 = 1.5 psi
(diastolic; approximate minimum pressure)

That means that blood pressure within normal range puts between 2.3 pounds of pressure per square inch on the vessels at its highest and 1.5 pounds of pressure per square inch at its lowest. It can be even more during exercise or periods of stress. That's a lot of force on the arteries.

Getting healthy often involves completely changing the way you live, eat, sleep, and move. Although there aren't immediate, visible results, you will eventually begin to see the effects of your great choices. In the meantime, your blood pressure readings and heart rate can give you a window into your progress. As you continue your healthy habits for days, weeks, months, years, and the rest of your life, you're making the best choices you can to live vitally as you age.

In combination with the healthy lifestyle we just discussed, supplementation can be your biggest ally in preventing or reversing endothelial dysfunction—and, as a result, CVD. The next pages take an in-depth look at 10 Power Nutrients to support the health of your endothelium.

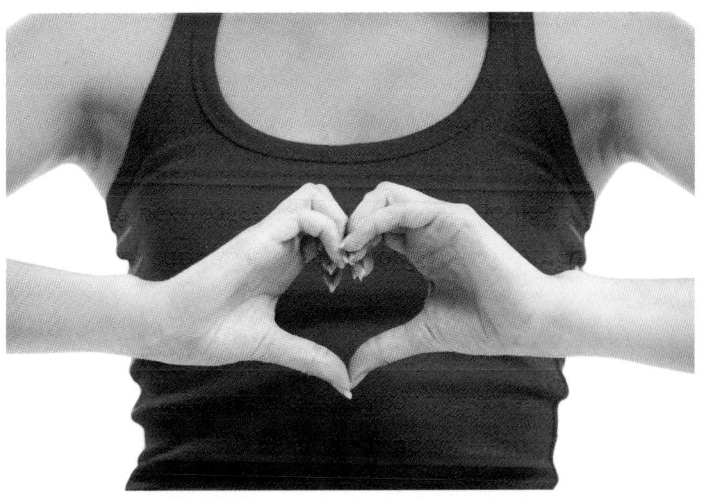

10 Power Nutrients to Support Endothelial Health

Supplements are a powerful tool for supporting endothelial health; it's important to note, however, that they are designed to supplement a healthy nutritional lifestyle, not replace it. The better your diet, the more benefits you'll receive from the supplements you take. Whether in a powder, capsule, shake, or liquid, supplements make it convenient and affordable to make sure you're getting all the nutrients you need to maintain total health and target the health of particular systems in the body. At their most basic, supplements simplify the process of getting nutrients.

Despite the powerful benefits, only slightly more than half of the US population takes supplements, according to the CDC. One reason is because there is limited education about the incredible healing effects nutrients can have on the body. Energy, vitality, improvement in mood, better sleep, improvement in muscle recovery after exercise, weight loss—these are all the results of a great lifestyle and targeted supplementation regimen. Supplements have such an important health impact, in fact, that findings published in the *Journal of the American Medical Association* (JAMA) stated that all adults should take daily vitamin supplements.

For some people, though, starting supplementation can feel overwhelming. Just walk into the supplement section of any major store, and you can instantly see why. There are so many options to choose from—how can a person sort through them all, let alone select the right supplements for their specific needs?

Compound that with the fact that supplements take a long time to show their effects (see "Reframing the Approach," page 74, for an in-depth discussion on why). Supplementing can't be thought of in terms of days, weeks, or months; it must be thought of in terms of *years* and *decades*. Each of those days, weeks, months, years, and decades add up to a lifetime of wellness and vitality.

Those three issues—lack of education surrounding the power of nutrients, the overwhelming feeling often experienced while selecting nutrients, and the difficulty of measuring progress—are exactly why we've identified 10 Power Nutrients that you can take to keep your endothelium in peak form. To help record and identify improvement as you get healthier, be sure to read the previous section, "Measuring Your Progress," which details how to track your blood pressure.

Getting Started with Supplements

The human body is complex and needs a wide array of nutrients to function optimally. Your needs are unique and specific. That's because no two people are exactly alike or put the exact same stressors on their body.

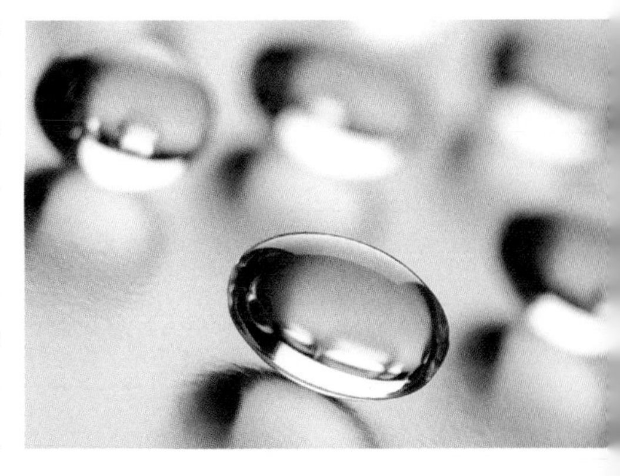

One way of knowing whether you're getting adequate nutrition is through a blood test. Based on the results, an expert in naturopathic medicine or a knowledgeable health care provider could put together a supplementation plan perfectly suited to your needs. But we realize getting a blood test is not practical or available for everyone. Our goal is to get you started with the basics, but keep in mind that we can't replace the advice of a nutrition expert who has the opportunity to sit down and talk with you about your lifestyle and needs. We'll provide a great start, but it's important to find someone you trust to help you build a program. You have to begin somewhere, and we'll give recommendations to get you started.

Before you begin supplementing with the 10 Power Nutrients in this next section, be sure you've built your nutritional base, including supplements to support total health. Along with a healthy diet, start with a multivitamin, an Omega-3 supplement, vitamin D, and CoQ10, and then add supplements that target the specific concerns you have. As you shop for your supplements, look for combination products that contain several nutrients; they're combined to make it easier for you to quickly get several nutrients at once. Instead of taking fifteen supplements, for example, you might only need to take four.

The next section details a plan that will help you deliver all of the key nutrients your endothelium needs to function optimally, produce more NO, and release all of those vital chemicals, hormones, and molecules into the body. Keep in mind that our recommended dosages are for adults. Children and adults who are taking medications or have a health concern should talk to their health care providers to determine a healthy intake of the 10 Power Nutrients.

10 Power Nutrients

1. **Amino acids: L-arginine, L-citrulline, L-taurine**
2. **Antioxidants: vitamin C, alpha lipoic acid, pomegranate, Pycnogenol®, resveratrol, grape seed/skin extract**
3. **Vitamin D3**
4. **Omega-3 fatty acids: fish oil, krill oil, and algal (vegan) sources**
5. **Omega-7 fatty acids**
6. **CoQ10**
7. **Green tea extract**
8. **Cocoa extract**
9. **Chromium picolinate**
10. **Garlic**

The moment you begin making positive lifestyle changes and start giving your endothelium the 10 Power Nutrients it needs to function optimally is the same moment you start repairing the endothelial cells and reversing cardiovascular dysfunction. The very first day you change your habits is the start of a new, healthy life. Supplements aren't a cure. But, in combination with a healthy diet and regular exercise, they might be the little bit extra you need to reverse CVD and save your life.

Amino Acids: L-Arginine, L-Citrulline, L-Taurine

You've likely seen food labels touting amino acids, and many probably listed health benefits. But what those labels probably didn't say is that, without amino acids, you couldn't stay alive. Proteins are made up of amino acids; once the body breaks down proteins, amino acids are left over. The nutrients are required for basic life functions. Without them, your body wouldn't be able to heal and regenerate tissues, grow, break down and digest food, and perform a number of other functions. Basically, your body wouldn't work.

When it comes to the endothelium, there are three amino acids that are absolutely crucial: L-arginine, L-citrulline, and L-taurine. L-arginine is the main nutrient source that supports the endothelium's ability to produce NO; L-citrulline and L-taurine both support L-arginine's role in promoting NO production. Multiple studies have shown L-arginine's ability to increase vasodilation in the blood vessels, including one study in the *International Journal of Cardiology*, which showed that supplemental L-arginine improved dilation of the brachial (upper arm) artery in patients with essential hypertension. A separate study in *The Journal of Clinical Investigation* found that a deficiency in L-arginine caused endothelial dysfunction due to decreased NO production in their study subjects. And yet another article published in *Circulation* identified that long-term supplemental L-arginine improves coronary small-vessel endothelial function, and that L-arginine may be a "therapeutic option for patients with coronary endothelial dysfunction and nonobstructive coronary artery disease." Since L-citrulline and L-taurine are needed for L-arginine to do its job well, all three are crucial to maintaining the health of the endothelium.

While adding food rich in L-arginine seems to be the best way to increase intake, there's a catch: after consuming the nutrient, only about 40 percent makes it to the endothelium and other areas in the body. The other 60 percent is metabolized. Plus, only about 5 percent of the average adult's diet includes L-arginine, which is not enough for optimal function. We've found that supplementing with the amino acids L-arginine, L-citrulline, and L-taurine is the only way to ensure you're getting enough of these necessary nutrients to keep the endothelium healthy and NO levels at their peak. **Recommended dosage: L-arginine, 5,000 milligrams (mg) per day; L-citrulline, 500 to 2,000 mg per day; L-taurine, 2,000 mg per day**

Antioxidants: Vitamin C, Alpha Lipoic Acid, Pomegranate, Pycnogenol®, Resveratrol, Grape Seed/Skin Extract

We've already discussed free radicals and antioxidants at length, so we won't repeat ourselves (see page 47 for a recap). But we would like to reiterate a key point: antioxidants help combat damage to the endothelium. They're critical to keeping the endothelial cells healthy so they can secrete the necessary chemicals, hormones, and molecules needed to keep the blood vessels smooth and flexible. A scientific review from Boston University School of Medicine concluded, "Considerable data also indicates that antioxidant compounds limit oxidative damage and restore endothelial function." When antioxidants decline, so does the health of the endothelium. Similarly, when you flood your endothelium with antioxidants, it supports the natural regenerative process of the endothelial cells.

There are numerous antioxidants that support endothelial health, but we've narrowed it to six:

- **Vitamin C**—Vitamin C is one of the only nutrients that has an immediate effect on the endothelium; in fact, taking vitamins C and E before eating a high-fat meal can even protect the body from temporary endothelial impairment. Research published in *Circulation* showed that both single-dose and long-term supplementation with vitamin C increases the production of NO. A low level of C has also been associated with increased inflammation and an impaired vascular system in lean and obese men. **Recommended dosage: 1,000 to 2,000 milligrams (mg) per day**

- **Alpha lipoic acid (ALA)**—A placebo-controlled study of thirty people with Type 2 diabetes found that treatment with intravenous ALA improved blood vessel dilation. Other findings published in *Free Radical Biology and Medicine* found that ALA has therapeutic potential for people with diabetes. Our experience shows that ALA is an important antioxidant in improving endothelial function. **Recommended dosage: 300 to 600 milligrams (mg) per day**

- **Pomegranate**—More than just a delicious snack or drink, pomegranate is one of the most powerful antioxidants for supporting endothelial health. Research in *Atherosclerosis* demonstrated that pomegranate juice not only reverses atherosclerosis but can also protect against CVD, in part due to the juice lowering the impact of oxidative stress. Pomegranate extract concentrates the benefits of the fruit into capsule form. **Recommended dosage: Juice, 8 to 16 ounces of 100 percent pomegranate juice per day; supplement, natural pomegranate polyphenol extract (standardized to 30 percent punicalagins), 1,000 milligrams (mg) per day**

- **Pycnogenol®**—An extract from the bark of French maritime pine trees, Pycnogenol® is a potent antioxidant, has natural anti-inflammatory properties, and encourages the production of NO. It's best known for its cardiovascular benefits, including prevention of atherosclerosis. Findings published in *Hypertension Research* showed that the extract boosts vasodilation through increased NO production and would be useful in treating diseases that stem from endothelial dysfunction. **Recommended dosage: 100 to 200 milligrams (mg) per day**

- **Resveratrol**—Resveratrol, a polyphenol found in red wine and other plant sources, has antioxidant properties that have been shown to be heart-healthy. A study in *Arteriosclerosis, Thrombosis, and Vascular Biology* found that the nutrient improves endothelial function in people with Type 2 diabetes. And an article in *Cardiovascular Drugs and Therapy* adds that resveratrol boosts NO production, and "accumulating reports have shown that resveratrol can prevent or slow the progression of a wide variety of diseases, including cancer, cardiovascular disease, ischemic injuries and Alzheimer's disease." **Recommended dosage: 100 to 200 milligrams (mg) per day**

- **Grape seed/skin extract**—Grapes have medicinal roots dating back nearly six thousand years to ancient Egypt. Today, antioxidant-rich grape seed and skin extract is used for a variety of health purposes, including supporting cardiovascular health. Research conducted at Boston University School of Medicine showed that purple grape extract inhibits platelet aggregation (platelet stickiness that can lead to clots) and increases NO production. **Recommended dosage: 50 to 100 milligrams (mg) per day**

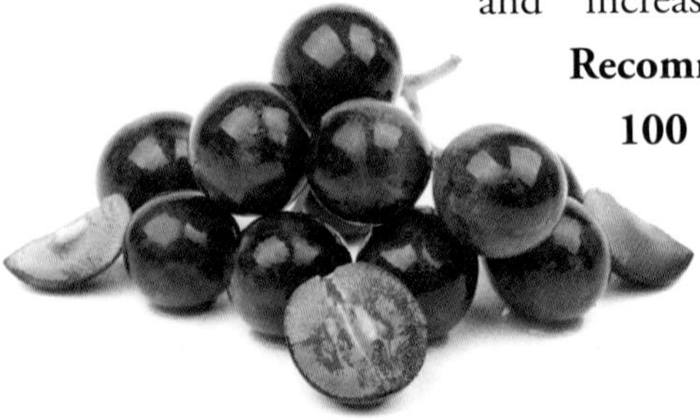

Vitamin D3

You've probably heard about the "sunshine vitamin," vitamin D3, which is the active form of vitamin D. The term comes from the best source of the nutrient: the sun. When sunlight shines on the skin, vitamin D is converted to vitamin D3, which our bodies use for a number of processes. Vitamin D3 is the active form, which maintains normal blood levels, as well as aids in bone absorption of calcium and phosphorus. Since most people are exposed to the sun almost every day, you'd think everyone would be getting enough of this critical nutrient. But a study in the journal *Nutrition Research* found that approximately 42 percent of the US population is not getting adequate vitamin D intake. And this number is even higher in the older population.

Deficiencies in D have been linked to all sorts of chronic diseases. According to the Harvard School of Public Health, D deficiency may increase the risk of certain cancers, osteoporosis, and infectious diseases like tuberculosis and the flu. What's most concerning to us is the impact of vitamin D on the endothelium and cardiovascular system.

Research in the journal *Circulation* found that deficiency in the vitamin can lead to CVD, including heart failure, hypertension (high blood pressure), and ischemic heart disease (reduced blood flow to the heart). Low levels of vitamin D can increase inflammation, which can cause endothelial dysfunction. Additional research published in *Hypertension* found that, when vitamin D levels are low, the endothelial cells produce proinflammatory substances.

On the reverse side, ample D has an anti-inflammatory effect in the cardiovascular system, reducing the chronic inflammation that puts wear on the endothelium.

According to the nonprofit organization The Vitamin D Council, exposing your bare skin to the sun for less than half the amount of time it takes your skin to turn pink should give you plenty of vitamin D. The amount of sun exposure needed varies drastically by skin type, time of day, and geographic location, ranging anywhere from six minutes to two hours. The Council also explains that you cannot get adequate vitamin D intake from food alone.

But even some people who get plenty of sunshine have low vitamin D levels. There are a number of reasons for this. Sunscreen, which "screens" the sun from your skin, blocks harmful UV rays but also keeps the skin from absorbing vitamin D. Long sleeves, hats, and other sun-protective clothing also blocks the sun's beneficial properties.

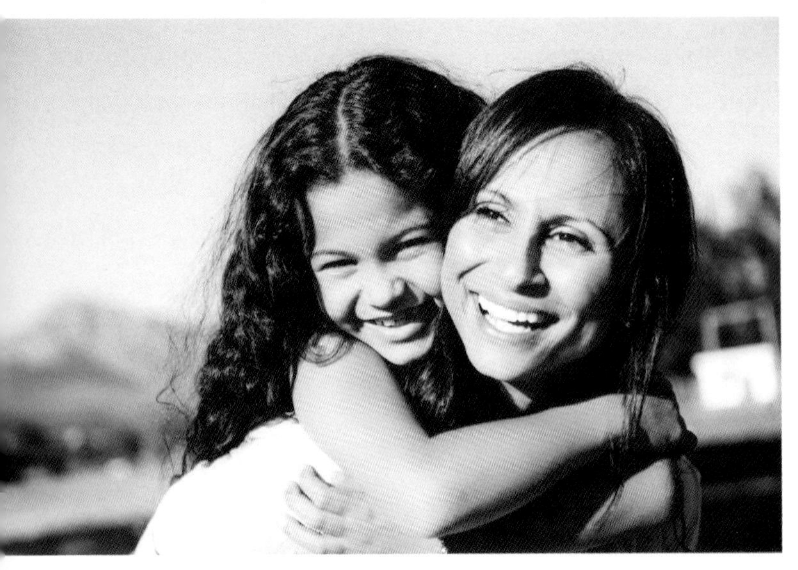

Furthermore, some people have trouble absorbing the nutrient because of other issues in the body like gut, kidney, or liver dysfunction. Even otherwise healthy people sometimes need much higher levels of the vitamin because their bodies have trouble absorbing and processing the nutrient. That's exactly why we recommend adding vitamin D to a healthy-endothelium supplementation regimen. **Recommended dosage: 2,000 to 5,000 International Units (IU) per day for adults and 10,000 IU per day for certain medical conditions. Consult your health care provider for appropriate blood work after ninety days of taking vitamin D3.**

Omega-3 Fatty Acids: Fish Oil, Krill Oil, and Algal (Vegan) Sources

Omega-3 fatty acids DHA and EPA have such a critical role in heart health that the American Heart Association recommends eating fatty fish twice per week. Even conventional medicine has accepted Omega-3s as an important part of preventing or reversing heart disease, with its key benefit in reducing inflammation. According to the Mayo Clinic, Omega-3s may lower triglycerides and blood pressure, reduce blood clotting, improve immunity, reduce symptoms of arthritis, and even improve learning ability in children. A meta-analysis of published research also found that supplementing with Omega-3 fatty acids "significantly improves endothelial function."

In supplement form, Omega-3s are available through fish oil, krill oil (from the shrimp-like crustacean krill), and algal (vegan, from algae) sources. One study found that supplemental fish oil significantly improved endothelial function and reduced inflammation in people with Type 2 diabetes. Researchers add that the fish oil "may have beneficial cardiovascular and metabolic health effects in otherwise healthy subjects predisposed to diabetes and its vascular complications."

Food sources like fish are a great way to get Omega-3 fatty acids DHA and EPA. Even with dietary fish consumption, though, an Omega-3 supplement is recommended. If you're vegan or vegetarian or can't handle the fishy aftertaste of some supplements, an algal (vegan) supplement might be your best choice. **Recommended dosage: 900 milligrams (mg) of EPA/DHA per day**

Omega-7 Fatty Acids

You've heard of Omega-3s and maybe even Omega-6s. But it's likely this is the first time you're hearing about heart-healthy Omega-7s. Omega-7 is a fatty acid found predominately in macadamia nut oil, fish oil, and sea buckthorn. While all are great sources of the fatty acid, purified forms from fish oil are free of palmitic acid, high levels of which are known to be toxic to the body.

Like better-known Omega-3 fatty acids, Omega-7s support the health of the endothelium and cardiovascular system. Preliminary studies indicate that purified Omega-7 from fish oil lowers levels of C-reactive protein. Elevations in C-reactive protein levels indicate inflammation in the endothelium and arterial wall. Reductions in C-reactive protein levels parallel decreases in inflammation, which lowers your risk for endothelial dysfunction, CVD, and stroke. Additional research shows that purified Omega-7 from fish oil may decrease insulin resistance, lower blood sugar, and decrease triglyceride and LDL cholesterol levels, while increasing good HDL levels.

While research on purified Omega-7s is still emerging, studies have explored the benefits of sea buckthorn oil and macadamia nut oil. According to a review in the *Journal of Ethnopharmacology*, the fruit and leaves of sea buckthorn "are well known to improve the functioning of the cardiovascular system." Sea buckthorn also has antiatherogenic effects, meaning it helps prevent atherosclerosis (hardening of the arteries), according to the authors. Other research published in the *Journal of Cardiovascular Pharmacology* showed that sea buckthorn protects the endothelial cells from injuries resulting from oxidized LDL ("bad") cholesterol and also helps maintain endothelial function.

Scientists at Pennsylvania State University also found that a diet rich in macadamia nuts reduces total and LDL cholesterol in people with mildly high blood cholesterol levels. LDL cholesterol is one of the five "highs" (see page 57), so reducing LDL is an important part of supporting endothelial function. You can increase your Omega-7 intake by eating macadamia nuts, or opt for a purified Omega-7 fish oil supplement. **Recommended dosage: 420 to 840 milligrams (mg) per day**

CoQ10

Coenzyme Q10, or CoQ10, is a necessary component in the process of converting food into energy, and it also aids in cell growth and repair. CoQ10 must be present in the mitochondria, a specialized structure in the cells that facilitates energy production, for the food you eat to be converted into energy. The organ with the largest concentration of mitochondria? The heart. So, it's especially critical that the heart receives plenty of CoQ10.

The coenzyme is also a powerful antioxidant that helps reduce the impact of free radicals on the endothelium (for more on oxidation and free radicals, see page 47). Research conducted by the European Society of Cardiology suggests that supplementing with CoQ10 may help patients with endothelial dysfunction by counteracting NO oxidation. The coenzyme additionally helps prevent LDL cholesterol oxidation and promotes optimal cell function. It can also improve endothelial function in patients with Type 2 diabetes who are taking statins, according to a study in *Diabetes Care*.

While the nutrient has several cardio-supportive benefits, it's best known for its ability to reverse atherosclerosis (see page 47 for more on atherosclerosis). One study conducted by Los Angeles Biomedical Research Institute found that a combination of CoQ10 and aged garlic "reduced the progression of coronary atherosclerosis." We'll add that it doesn't just stop progression—it reverses it. Because the coenzyme supports the individual endothelial cells and has an antioxidant effect on the endothelium, it also enhances the endothelium's ability to restore function so the arteries become more flexible.

A meta-analysis of several studies nicely reiterates our point: "Coenzyme Q10 supplementation is associated with significant improvement in endothelial function." The review also mentions that current research supports CoQ10's role in treating endothelial dysfunction. If you're looking to prevent or reverse heart disease, CoQ10 is an excellent endothelium-supportive nutrient. **Recommended dosage: 200 to 400 milligrams (mg) per day**

Green Tea Extract

Tea isn't just a refreshing or comforting beverage—it's loaded with all kinds of health benefits. With tea second only to water as the most widely consumed beverage in the world, it's encouraging to know a favorite drink is good for you, too. Dried tea leaves contain many wellness-enhancing nutrients, and green tea extract is especially great for the endothelium.

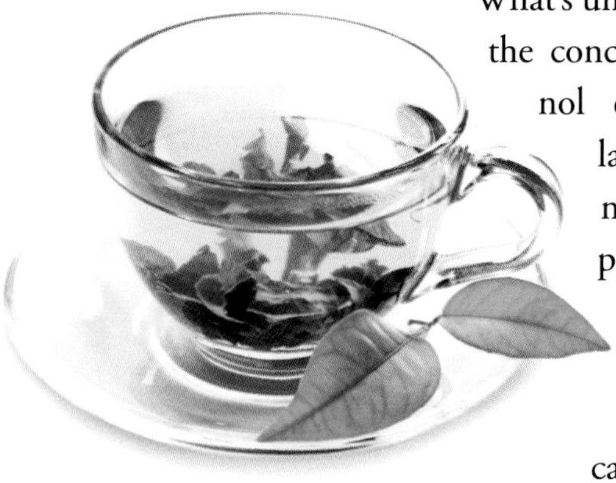

What's unique about green tea is the concentration of polyphenol epigallocatechin-3-gallate (EGCG) and flavonoids. Polyphenols are powerful antioxidants that help prevent atherosclerosis by helping reduce free radical damage and prevent LDL cholesterol oxidation. Flavonoids are a subclass of polyphenols and are produced in plants. They are the colors in fruits and vegetables that protect plants from disease. In plants—and in us—they function as antioxidants.

According to a research overview in the *Journal of the American College of Nutrition*, "epidemiological and intervention studies indicate that consumption of 5–6 or more cups of green tea, containing 200–300 mg EGCG, per day may be beneficial for maintaining cardiovascular and metabolic health." Another study in the *American Journal of Physiology: Endocrinology and Metabolism* found that the benefits of ECGC on the cardiovascular and metabolic systems may be from the nutrient stimulating NO production.

The flavonoids in green tea are also incredibly beneficial to the endothelial cells and cardiovascular system. An article in *Molecular Aspects of Medicine* states that "there is now consistent data indicating that tea and tea flavonoids can enhance nitric oxide status and improve endothelial function." Getting adequate intake of the flavonoids significantly lowers your risk of cancer, CVD, and many other health issues.

Green tea has been used for centuries to promote health and prevent disease. Thankfully, you can get the benefits of several cups of the healthful drink in just one tablet. **Recommended dosage: 100 milligrams (mg) per day**

Cocoa (Bean) Extract

Cocoa is one of our favorite Power Nutrients. Not only is it delicious, but it's also extremely healthful. Extract from the cocoa plant contains polyphenols, particularly the flavonoid subclass flavanols, which are antioxidants that stimulate NO production and combat free radical damage to the endothelial cells. While the nutrient is known for lowering blood pressure and increasing circulation, the core benefit is to the endothelium.

A study at UC Davis found that cocoa activates the endothelium to produce NO, which signals the smooth muscle wall to relax, or widen. Research published in *Hypertension* found that cocoa can lower blood pressure, increase endothelium-dependent vasodilation, and reduce insulin resistance in people with essential hypertension. Findings from a study at the Yale Prevention Research Center also demonstrated that liquid cocoa and solid dark chocolate can improve endothelial function and reduce blood pressure in overweight adults. And research published in the *Journal of the American College of Cardiology* states: "Diets rich in flavanols reverse vascular dysfunction in diabetes, highlighting therapeutic potentials in cardiovascular disease."

There are multiple other studies that detail the benefits of cocoa, especially in people with advanced dysfunction like diabetes or CVD. But it's important to remember that anyone can benefit from the nutrient. Cocoa supports endothelial health by helping maintain what's already healthy and repair what's not.

Supplemental cocoa extract concentrates the power of the antioxidant-rich cocoa plant, often yielding the benefits of an entire chocolate bar without the added fats, sugars, and high calorie intake. Also, some of the flavanols can be damaged in the process of making chocolate, so extract can often deliver greater health benefits than solid chocolate. So, enjoy dark chocolate in moderation, but consider adding a cocoa (bean) extract containing cocoa flavonols to your Power Nutrient regimen. **Recommended dosage: 900 milligrams (mg) per day**

Chromium Picolinate

Chromium is an essential trace element in the human body and is involved in a number of physiological processes. The supplemental form known as chromium picolinate has been shown to lower blood sugar, increase effectiveness of insulin, reduce high blood pressure, aid weight loss, improve symptoms of diabetes, prevent heart disease, and restore endothelial health.

Several studies confirm the effectiveness of dietary chromium and make a case for supplementation. According to a scientific review by *Harvard Health Publications*, along with a healthy diet and regular exercise, chromium may boost HDL ("good") cholesterol; recall that low HDL is one of the five "highs" that contribute to endothelial dysfunction (see page 57). The publication also notes that low levels of chromium have been associated with higher incidence of heart attack. The article further explains, "Since chromium influences insulin action and glucose metabolism, diabetes is a logical candidate for chromium replacement therapy." Many of the symptoms associated with diabetes also put wear and stress on the endothelium, making chromium supplementation an important part of reversing endothelial dysfunction, especially in people with diabetes.[1]

Chromium is found in whole-grain breads and cereals, lean meats, oatmeal, mushrooms, asparagus, and nuts, among other sources. If you're having a hard time getting enough chromium in your diet—or if you're dealing with metabolic syndrome or diabetes—you might consider adding supplementary chromium, known as chromium picolinate. **Recommended dosage: 400 to 1,000 micrograms (mcg) per day**

Garlic

The same herb that adds flavor to pasta sauce and gives New York-style pizza its kick is also great for your health. Consuming high amounts of garlic has been linked to decreased cancer rates, lower cholesterol levels, and lower risk

1 If you are diabetic and taking medications or insulin, check with your health care provider regarding your use of chromium picolinate.

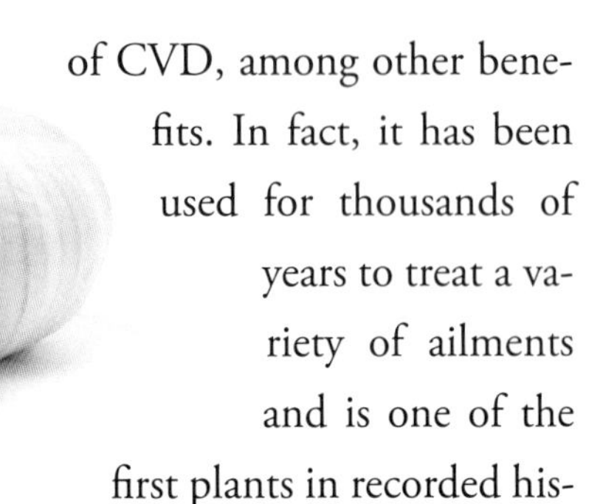

of CVD, among other benefits. In fact, it has been used for thousands of years to treat a variety of ailments and is one of the first plants in recorded history that was used for maintaining health and treating disease. It was even used in ancient Greece as a "performance enhancer" for athletes in the Olympic Games! Now, more and more research is being done on this herb to understand how it works in the body.

According to research conducted at the University of Alabama at Birmingham, this super food increases the body's natural production of hydrogen sulfide, a signaling antioxidant that is involved in relaxing blood vessels and increasing blood flow. Later research published in *Frontiers in Physiology* showed that hydrogen sulfide is involved with the regulation of NO production in the endothelial cells and that hydrogen sulfide deficiencies may impact NO levels. So, garlic stimulates the production of hydrogen sulfide, which acts as a vascular cell signaling molecule and stimulates the endothelial cells to produce NO, which causes the blood vessels to relax and blood to flow better through the vessels, and has a host of other healthful benefits within the cardiovascular system. The herb is also a strong antioxidant that helps reduce the impact of free radicals on the endothelial cells.

Aged garlic extract has been extensively researched, as well. While fresh garlic gives a strong odor from the compound allicin, aged garlic does not. One study in *Phytotherapy Research* showed that supplementing with aged garlic extract improved endothelial function in men with coronary artery disease who were taking statins and aspirin. Its major benefit? It acts as an antioxidant and has an anti-inflammatory effect in the endothelial cells, as well as increases the body's natural production of NO. Other studies have shown the extract's ability to not only slow or stop plaque buildup but possibly also reverse buildup that has already occurred. And findings published in the *Journal of Nutrition* state that "...compelling evidence supports the beneficial health effects attributed to [aged garlic extract, including] reducing the risk of cardiovascular disease, stroke, cancer and aging, including the oxidant-mediated brain cell damage that is implicated in Alzheimer's disease."

Here's the catch: to get the great benefits of fresh garlic, you would need to eat between two and twelve medium-sized cloves a day. Of course, the best source is always diet, and we encourage you to try to get your intake through whole food sources. But if you're like us and struggle to work large amounts of fresh garlic into your meals, a supplement might be a great option. Most aged garlic supplements will pack the nutritional benefits of an entire clove of garlic in just one capsule—without the after-smell the potent plant can have on your sweat and breath. **Recommended dosage: 600 to 1,200 milligrams (mg) per day, or the equivalent of one to two cloves**

We've spent countless hours poring over scientific studies, identifying the 10 Power Nutrients most critical to the endothelium and cardiovascular system as a whole. We then took all of that material and distilled it into a readable and accessible form, giving you the knowledge you need to be well. Each nutrient plays a specific role in supporting the health of the endothelium. While they might have similar functions—stimulating NO, for example—each serves a unique purpose in supporting endothelial health. And remember: the endothelium can only be healthy if your body is healthy. Building a nutritional food base that emphasizes the foods found in the Mediterranean diet is the first step. Then, as you're building or maintaining that nutritional base, we recommend adding in the 10 Power Nutrients to more fully support endothelial health.

Putting It All Together

Supporting and maintaining a lifetime of endothelial health depends on a holistic approach that must include all aspects of your lifestyle. Promoting endothelial function will improve your overall health, longevity, and vitality, while also directly reducing your risk of degenerative diseases like heart disease and stroke.

We know it can seem overwhelming to completely shift your mind-set and change your life for the better. To help, we've put together a simple plan for endothelial health, meant to help you build an individualized plan of your own. We hope our recommendations will help you begin a journey toward a healthier cardiovascular system and better life:

Be happy. Build your life around happiness and gratitude. Happiness is the experience of joy, contentment, and positive well-being, combined with a sense that one's life is good, meaningful, and worthwhile.

Relax. Use daily breathing exercises to help reduce the impact of stressors on your mind and body. A minimum of five minutes a day of mindful breathing can help to offset the damaging effects of stress.

Eat fresh. Focus your diet around fresh, local, whole fruits and vegetables. Choose healthy protein options and limit your intake of all the bad foods that are so prevalent in today's standard American diet—processed foods, fast foods, and saturated and trans fats.

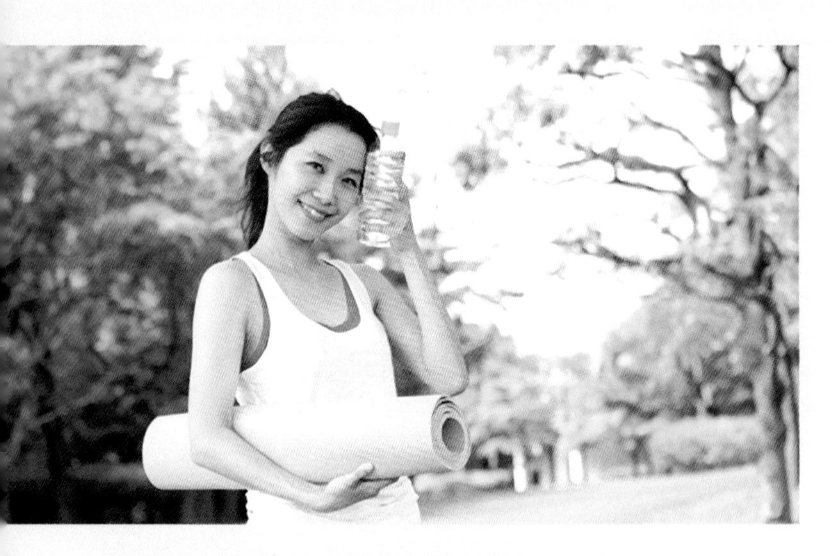

Drink more water. Hydration plays a tremendous role in overall endothelial health and function. Maintaining your daily intake of water is critically important to overall health and bodily functions, and your endothelium is especially thirsty. Make water your first choice of beverages, and be consistent with your intake.

Get plenty of sleep. Optimizing your sleep habits will do wonders for your overall health and especially your endothelium. Sleep is an underrated promoter of health, and more and more research indicates that those who are sleep-deprived face greater risk for CVD. Eight or more hours of sleep on a consistent basis will support the repair and regenerative mechanisms of the body and promote endothelial function.

Exercise regularly. We've provided numerous examples of the benefits of exercise in the promotion of endothelial health. Your commitment to regular, daily exercise is one of the best ways to boost your NO production and optimal endothelial health.

Maintain nutritional support. Even with a great diet, the addition of supplemental nutrition is critical to optimizing your endothelial health and function over your lifetime. In addition to a daily multivitamin, we recommend the following targeted Power Nutrients as part of a supplement program for total endothelial health and NO optimization. We recommend starting with the following daily targeted regimen:[1]

L-arginine	5,000 mg
L-citrulline	500 to 2,000 mg
Omega-3 fatty acids	900 mg EPA/DHA
Vitamin D	2,000 to 5,000 IU
Antioxidant nutrients; examples include:	1,000 to 2,000 mg of vitamin C
	300 to 600 mg of Alpha Lipoic Acid (ALA)
CoQ10	200 to 400 mg
Omega-7	420 to 840 mg
Green tea extract	100 mg
Chromium picolinate	400 to 1,000 mcg

For a convenient, printable list of our 10 Power Nutrients, including dosages, please visit HealthIsWealth.net.

1 There are several other nutrients discussed in Section 3. For additional options, please review the individual nutrients.

Conclusion

Do you now feel like an expert in endothelial health? You should. You've learned information that some of the most renowned cardiovascular specialists don't even know. Knowledge is power. This knowledge can save lives. Not just yours, but anyone who's willing to listen to the message of endothelial health we've just shared with you.

We've spent pages exploring a complex and unique organ known as the endothelium. It's complex because it extends throughout the entire body, lining one hundred thousand miles of blood vessels and protecting the smooth muscle of the arteries. It's unique because it not only completely reframes everything we know about organs, but it also has an incredible role in every system of the body. Our discussion has focused on the vascular endothelium and its function within the heart, arteries, veins, and capillaries. And because our focus has been narrowed to the cardiovascular system, and primarily the arteries within that system, we've only skimmed the surface of this complex organ.

What's most fascinating to us about endothelial cells is that they change function as they move into different systems of the body. While it's one continuous, communicative organ, the role of the endothelium is unique to the given organ it's working in, near, or around. That means that the endothelial cells in the kidney excrete different substances than the endothelial cells in the cardiovascular system. Some of the chemicals, hormones, and molecules it produces are the same—NO, for example—but the individual endothelial cells adapt to meet the demands of the system (kidney, liver, or digestive tract, for example) they're in.

Nutrients and botanicals also impact the endothelium's many functions differently. Take the brain, for example. Botanicals like the herb ginkgo biloba have specific components that target the health of the endothelial cells in the brain. Research in *Cellular and Molecular Life Sciences* found that gingko biloba affects blood flow to the brain and NO levels.

Nutrients have an affinity for certain *types* of endothelial cells. Incredible! Think of the research potential. Think of the potential for human health. Think of the potential for preventing and reversing disease...and saving lives.

While there have been extensive studies proving that the endothelium is the base for cardiovascular health, research on endothelial cells in the rest the body is still new. We're excited about the therapeutic opportunities available by studying the endothelium's role in other systems. What if the endothelium is the base of *all* health? What if the plaque that causes Alzheimer's is really endothelial dysfunction?

What if plaque in the brain could be reversed like plaque in the arteries? Sure, the brain is different—cells don't regenerate like they do in the cardiovascular system—but what if diseases like Alzheimer's could literally be stopped in their tracks?

We expect researchers to find that the endothelium is just as powerful in other systems as it is in the cardiovascular system. We anxiously await the day when these discoveries are made.

For now, though, there is a story to share: the story of the endothelium. We are firmly convinced, and scientific studies have confirmed, that understanding the endothelium is the key to changing the statistics on CVD. If everyone understands the power of the endothelium, and puts into practice the strategies in this book, just imagine what could happen. Imagine a world where everyone lives vitally well into their advanced years—where people seventy, eighty, and even ninety years old lead complete and fulfilling lives free from disease.

The potential is there. But it takes thousands and millions of voices to spread the story. You are an important part in spreading the message; together, we can make a difference. Will you join your voice with ours?

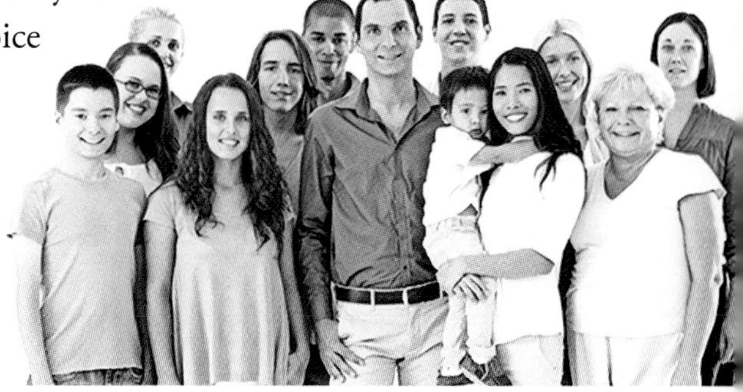

Acknowledgments

It takes many supportive people to give life to a concept and book like *The New Heart Health.* To each and every person who has been a part of the development of this book, we would like to offer a humble and heartfelt, "Thank you!"

Thank you, as well, to the readers of this book who believe that "health care is really self-care" and are willing to help share our wellness message with their families, friends, and coworkers. We wrote *The New Heart Health* for the purpose of empowering our readers to take charge of their own wellness and make a positive and lasting impact on their quality of life.

Our deepest thanks also go to:

Our families and friends for their constant love and support throughout the book development process.

Our friend and business partner, Dave Brubaker, whose entrepreneurial spirit helps to guide our success.

Our internal book production and online team: Stacy Ennis for her amazing writing skills and coordination of the book project; Landon Wackerli for his project management and the expansion of the *Health Is Wealth* concept and brand; Karen McGinty for jumping in and making things happen on all ends of the project; Kelly Cope for her leadership and organizational skills; Shannon Tracy for her research, support, and keeping up with the health science side of this project; Amy Meyer for her constant support and dedicated hard work; Shiloh Schroeder for cover design, layout, and graphics; Karen McGinty, Kim Foster, and Robin Bethel for proofreading and final polishing of our content; and Tami Bosworth for additional graphic support. And a special thanks to Dr. James Hollingsworth for his hard work and medical expertise in the review and editing process; Gary Amato for his management and negotiation skills; C&S Sales for distribution; and Creel Printing for printing and shipping.

References

Introduction

Yusuf, S., Hawken, S., Ounpuu, S., Dans, T., Avezum, A., Lanas, F., ... INTERHEART Study Investigators. (2004). Effect of potentially modifiable risk factors associated with myocardial infarction in 52 countries (the INTERHEART study): case-control study. *Lancet, 364* (9438), 11-17.

Larsen, P. O., & Ins, M. (2010). The rate of growth in scientific publication and the decline in coverage provided by Science Citation Index. *Scientometrics, 84* (3), 575-603.

National Library of Medicine (U.S.), & North, M. J. (2002). *Greek medicine: "I swear by Apollo physician": Greek medicine from the gods to Galen.* Bethesda, MD: National Library of Medicine, National Institutes of Health, Dept. of Health and Human Services.

Alonso-Zaldivar, R. (2011, July 28). Health care costs to account for one-fifth of U.S. economy by 2020: report. Retrieved from http://www.huffingtonpost.com/2011/07/28/health-care-costs-economy-us_n_911917.html

Section 1

WHO. Cardiovascular diseases (CVDs). (2013, March). Retrieved from http://www.who.int/mediacentre/factsheets/fs317/en/index.html

CDC. *Heart disease facts.* (n.d.). Retrieved from http://www.cdc.gov/heartdisease/facts.htm

WHO. 10 leading causes of death in females. (n.d.). Retrieved from http://www.who.int/gho/women_and_health/mortality/causes_death/en/index.html

Mayo Clinic. *Heart disease in women: Understand symptoms and risk factors* (n.d.). Retrieved from http://www.mayoclinic.com/health/heart-disease/HB00040

CDC. (n.d.). *Heart disease fact sheet.* Retrieved from http://www.cdc.gov/dhdsp/data_statistics/fact_sheets/docs/fs_heart_disease.pdf

CDC. (2013, May 30). *FASTSTATS - Heart disease.* Retrieved from http://www.cdc.gov/nchs/fastats/heart.htm

Cleaver, O., & Melton, D. A. (2003). Endothelial signaling during development. *Nature Medicine, 9* (6), 661-668.

Colman, J. (2005). Why our arteries become clogged as we age. *Life Extension Magazine, 2006.* Retrieved from http://www.lef.org/magazine/mag2005/dec2005_supp_atherosclerosis_01.htm?source=search&key=%22Maintaining%20the%20endotheliums%20integrity%20is%20crucial%20to%22

Section 2

WebMD. (n.d.). *Atherosclerosis overview* [Video file]. Retrieved from http://www.webmd.com/heart-disease/video/atherosclerosis

CDC. (2009). *The power of prevention.* Retrieved from http://www.cdc.gov/chronicdisease/pdf/2009-power-of-prevention.pdf

CDC. (2012, August 7). *Facts about physical activity.* Retrieved from http://www.cdc.gov/physicalactivity/data/facts.html

Lopez-Garcia, E., & Hu, F. B. (2004). Nutrition and the endothelium. *Current Diabetes Reports, 4 (*4), 253-259.

Sears, W. (2010). *Prime-time health.* New York, NY: Little, Brown and Company.

CDC. (2012, August 13). *Adult obesity facts.* Retrieved from http://www.cdc.gov/obesity/data/adult.htmlLife Extension (n.d.). *Atherosclerosis and Cardiovascular Disease.* Retrieved from http://www.lef.org/protocols/heart_circulatory/coronary_artery_disease_atherosclerosis_01.htm

Toikka, J. O., Ahotupa, M., Viikari, J. S. A., Niinikoski, H., Taskinen, M.-R., Irjala, K., Hartiala, J. J., (1999). Constantly low HDL-cholesterol concentration relates to endothelial dysfunction and increased in vivo LDL-oxidation in healthy young men. *Atherosclerosis, 147* (1), 133-138.

Haas, R. (2011). Widely used in Europe...Natural sedative restores youthful sleep. *Life Extension Magazine*, April 2011. Retrieved from http://www.lef.org/magazine/mag2011/apr2011_Widely-Used-in-Europe-Natural-Sedative-Restores-Youthful-Sleep_01.htm?source=search&key=cortisol%20sleep

Chumaeva, N. (2010, June 23). *Chronic and acute stress in atherosclerosis: The role of endothelial function and arterial elasticity.* Retrieved from https://helda.helsinki.fi/handle/10138/19839?show=full

Namtvedt, S. K., Hisdal, J., Randby, A., Agewall, S., Stranden, E., Somers, V. K., Røsjø, H., (2013). Impaired endothelial function in persons with obstructive sleep apnoea: Impact of obesity. *Heart, 99 (*1), 30-34.

Mayo Clinic. (2013, June 15). *Obstructive sleep apnea: Symptoms.* Retrieved from http://www.mayoclinic.com/health/obstructive-sleep-apnea/DS00968/DSECTION=symptoms

Colman, J. (2005). Why our arteries become clogged as we age. *Life Extension Magazine, 2006.* Retrieved from http://www.lef.org/magazine/mag2005/dec2005_supp_atherosclerosis_01.htm?source=search&key=age%20endothelium

Singhal, A. (2005). Endothelial dysfunction: Role in obesity-related disorders and the early origins of CVD. *The Proceedings of the Nutrition Society, 64 (*1), 15-22.

CDC. (2013, July 10). *Childhood Obesity Facts*. Retrieved from http://www.cdc.gov/healthyyouth/obesity/facts.htm

Hornig, B., Arakawa, N., Kohler, C., & Drexler, H. (1998). Vitamin C improves endothelial function of conduit arteries in patients with chronic heart failure. *Circulation, 97* (4), 363-368.

Section 3

Borek, C. (2001). Antioxidant health effects of aged garlic extract. *The Journal of Nutrition, 131.*

Crews, F. T., & Nixon, K. (January 01, 2003). Alcohol, neural stem cells, and adult neurogenesis. *Alcohol Research & Health: The Journal of the National Institute on Alcohol Abuse and Alcoholism, 27* (2), 197-204.

Mayo Clinic. (2013, June 14). *Mediterranean diet: A heart-healthy eating plan.* Retrieved from http://www.mayoclinic.com/health/mediterranean-diet/CL00011

Marin, C., Ramirez, R., Delgado-Lista, J., Yubero-Serrano, E. M., Perez-Martinez, P., Carracedo, J., ... Lopez-Miranda, J. (2011). Mediterranean diet reduces endothelial damage and improves the regenerative capacity of endothelium. *The American Journal of Clinical Nutrition, 93* (2), 267-274.

Alexopoulos, N., Vlachopoulos, C., Aznaouridis, K., Baou, K., Vasiliadou, C., Pietri, P., ... Stefanadis, C. (2008). The acute effect of green tea consumption on endothelial function in healthy individuals. *European Journal of Cardiovascular Prevention and Rehabilitation: Official Journal of the European Society of Cardiology, Working Groups on Epidemiology & Prevention and Cardiac Rehabilitation and Exercise Physiology, 15* (3), 300-305.

Nagaya, N., Yamamoto, H., Uematsu, M., Itoh, T., Nakagawa, K., Miyazawa, T., ... Miyatake, K. (2004). Green tea reverses endothelial dysfunction in healthy smokers. *Heart 90* (12), 1485-1486.

Kim, W., Jeong, M. H., Cho, S. H., Yun, J. H., Chae, H. J., Ahn, Y. K., ... Kang, J. C. (2006). Effect of green tea consumption on endothelial function and circulating endothelial progenitor cells in chronic smokers. *Circulation Journal: Official Journal of the Japanese Circulation Society, 70* (8), 1052-1057.

Life Extension. (n.d.). *Atherosclerosis and cardiovascular disease.* Retrieved from http://www.lef.org/protocols/heart_circulatory/coronary_artery_disease_atherosclerosis_02.htm

Faridi, Z., Njike, V. Y., Dutta, S., Ali, A., & Katz, D. L. (2008). Acute dark chocolate and cocoa ingestion and endothelial function: A randomized controlled crossover trial. *The American Journal of Clinical Nutrition, 88* (1), 58-63.

Tuttle, D. (2007). Pomegranate reverses atherosclerosis and slows the progression of prostate cancer. *Life Extension Magazine*, February 2007. Retrieved from http://www.lef.org/magazine/mag2007/feb2007_report_pomegranate_01.htm

Webb, A. J., Patel, N., Loukogeorgakis, S., Okorie, M., Aboud, Z., Misra, S., ... Ahluwalia, A. (2008). Acute blood pressure lowering, vasoprotective, and antiplatelet properties of dietary nitrate via bioconversion to nitrite. *Hypertension, 51 (*3), 784-790.

Harvard School of Public Health. (n.d.). *The benefits of physical activity.* Retrieved from http://www.hsph.harvard.edu/nutritionsource/staying-active-full-story/

Hummel, S. G., Fischer, A. J., Martin, S. M., Schafer, F. Q., & Buettner, G. R. (2006). Nitric oxide as a cellular antioxidant: A little goes a long way. *Free Radical Biology and Medicine, 40* (3), 501-506.

Katzmarzyk, P. T., & Lee, I. M. (2012). Sedentary behaviour and life expectancy in the USA: A cause-deleted life table analysis. *BMJ Open, 2*, 4.

Hellmich, N. (2009, January 22). Q&A: How to drop pounds with all-day activities, not exercise. *USA Today.* Retrieved from http://usatoday30.usatoday.com/news/health/weightloss/2009-01-21-fidget-activity_N.htm

American Heart Association. (2012, April 4). *Understanding blood pressure readings.* Retrieved from http://www.heart.org/HEARTORG/Conditions/HighBloodPressure/AboutHighBloodPressure/Understanding-Blood-Pressure-Readings_UCM_301764_Article.jsp

Gahche, J., & National Center for Health Statistics (U.S.). (2011). *Dietary supplement use among U.S. adults has increased since NHANES III (1988-1994).* Hyattsville, MD: U.S. Dept. of Health & Human Services,

Centers for Disease Control and Prevention, National Center for Health Statistics.

Council for Responsible Nutrition. (2002, June 20). *Harvard researchers publish JAMA articles recommending vitamin supplements for all adults.* Retrieved from http://www.crnusa.org/shellnr062002.html

MedlinePlus (2011, February 8). *Amino acids.* Retrieved from http://www.nlm.nih.gov/medlineplus/ency/article/002222.htm

Lekakis, J. P., Papathanassiou, S., Papaioannou, T. G., Papamichael, C. M., Zakopoulos, N., Kotsis, V., ... Stamatelopoulos, S. F. (2002). Oral L-arginine improves endothelial dysfunction in patients with essential hypertension. *International Journal of Cardiology, 86,* 2-3.

Kamada, Y., Nagaretani, H., Tamura, S., Ohama, T., Maruyama, T., Hiraoka, H., ... Matsuzawa, Y. (2001). Vascular endothelial dysfunction resulting from L-arginine deficiency in a patient with lysinuric protein intolerance. *The Journal of Clinical Investigation, 108* (5), 717-724.

Lerman, A., Burnett, J. C. J., Higano, S. T., McKinley, L. J., & Holmes, D. R. J. (1998). Long-term L-arginine supplementation improves small-vessel coronary endothelial function in humans. *Circulation, 97 (21), 2123-2128.*

Wu, G. (2013). *Amino acids: Biochemistry and nutrition.*

Schulz, E., Anter, E., & Keaney, J. F. J. (2004). Oxidative stress, antioxidants, and endothelial function. *Current Medicinal Chemistry, 11 (*9), 1093-1104.

Barclay, L. (n.d.). High dose vitamin C a new therapeutic approach. *Life Extension Magazine*, October 2006. Retrieved from http://www.lef.org/magazine/mag2006/oct2006_report_vitaminc_01.htm?source=search&key=vitamin%20C%20endothelial

Gokce, N., Keaney, J. F. J., Frei, B., Holbrook, M., Olesiak, M., Zachariah, B. J., ... Vita, J. A. (1999). Long-term ascorbic acid administration reverses endothelial vasomotor dysfunction in patients with coronary artery disease. *Circulation, 99 (*25), 3234-3240.

Mah, E., Matos, M. D., Kawiecki, D., Ballard, K., Guo, Y., Volek, J. S., & Bruno, R. S. (2011). Vitamin C status is related to proinflammatory responses and impaired vascular endothelial function in healthy, college-aged lean and obese men. *Journal of the American Dietetic Association, 111* (5), 737-743.

Heinisch, B. B., Francesconi, M., Mittermayer, F., Schaller, G., Gouya, G., Wolzt, M., & Pleiner, J. (2010). Alpha-lipoic acid improves vascular endothelial function in patients with type 2 diabetes: A placebo-controlled randomized trial. *European Journal of Clinical Investigation, 40* (2), 148-154.

Heitzer, T., Finckh, B., Albers, S., Krohn, K., Kohlschütter, A., & Meinertz, T. (2001). Beneficial effects of alpha-lipoic acid and ascorbic acid on endothelium-dependent, nitric oxide-mediated vasodilation in diabetic patients: Relation to parameters of oxidative stress. *Free Radical Biology & Medicine, 31* (1), 53-61.

Aviram, M., & Dornfeld, L. (2001). Pomegranate juice consumption inhibits serum angiotensin converting enzyme activity and reduces systolic blood pressure. *Atherosclerosis, 158* (1), 195-198.

Horphag Research. (n.d.). *About Pycnogenol®*. Retrieved from http://www.pycnogenol.com/about/pycnogenol®/

Liu, F., Lau, B. H., Peng, Q., & Shah, V. (2000). Pycnogenol protects vascular endothelial cells from beta-amyloid-induced injury. *Biological & Pharmaceutical Bulletin, 23* (6), 735-737.

Mayo Clinic. (2011, June 9). *Red wine, antioxidants and resveratrol: Good for your heart?* Retrieved from http://www.mayoclinic.com/health/red-wine/HB00089

Zhang, H., Zhang, J., Ungvari, Z., & Zhang, C. (2009). Resveratrol improves endothelial function: Role of TNF and vascular oxidative stress. *Arteriosclerosis Thrombosis and Vascular Biology*, *29*, 1164-1171. doi:10.1161/ATVBAHA.109.187146

Li, H., & Fèorstermann, U. (2010). Erratum to: Resveratrol: A multifunctional compound improving endothelial function. *Cardiovascular Drugs and Therapy*, 24, 1.

University of Maryland Medical Center (2011, January 25). *Grape seed.* Retrieved from http://umm.edu/health/medical/altmed/herb/grape-seed

Vitseva, O., Varghese, S., Chakrabarti, S., Folts, J. D., & Freedman, J. E. (2005). Grape seed and skin extracts inhibit platelet function and release of reactive oxygen intermediates. *Journal of Cardiovascular Pharmacology, 46* (4), 445-451.

Forrest, K. Y. Z., & Stuhldreher, W. L. (2011). Prevalence and correlates of vitamin D deficiency in US adults. *Nutrition Research, 31* (1), 48-54.

Nitta, K. (2011). Impact of vitamin D metabolism on cardiovascular disease. *International Journal of Clinical Medicine, 2* (5), 531-537.

Harvard School of Public Health. (n.d.). *Vitamin D and health.* Retrieved from http://www.hsph.harvard.edu/nutritionsource/vitamin-d/#vitamin-d-deficiency-a-global-concern

Judd, S. E., & Tangpricha, V. (2009). Vitamin D deficiency and risk for cardiovascular disease. *The American Journal of the Medical Sciences, 338* (1), 40-44.

Jablonski, K. L., Chonchol, M., Pierce, G. L., Walker, A. E., & Seals, D. R. (2011). 25-hydroxyvitamin D deficiency is associated with inflammation-linked vascular endothelial dysfunction in middle-aged and older adults. *Hypertension, 57* (1), 63-69.

Vitamin D Council. (n.d.). *How do I get the vitamin D my body needs?* Retrieved from http://www.vitamindcouncil.org/about-vitamin-d/how-do-i-get-the-vitamin-d-my-body-needs/

Mayo Clinic. (2010, December 21). *Omega-3 in fish: How eating fish helps your heart.* Retrieved from http://www.mayoclinic.com/health/omega-3/HB00087

Wang, Q., Liang, X., Wang, L., Lu, X., Huang, J., Cao, J., ... Gu, D. (2012). Effect of omega-3 fatty acids supplementation on endothelial function: A meta-analysis of randomized controlled trials. *Atherosclerosis, 221* (2), 536-543.

Rizza, S., Tesauro, M., Cardillo, C., Galli, A., Iantorno, M., Gigli, F., ... Lauro, D. (2009). Fish oil supplementation improves endothelial function in normoglycemic offspring of patients with type 2 diabetes. *Atherosclerosis, 206* (2), 569-574.

Smith, M. A. (n.d.). Omega-7 fatty acids decrease hunger. Retrieved from http://blog.lef.org/2013/04/omega-7-fatty-acids-decrease-hunger.html

Suryakumar, G., & Gupta, A. (2011). Medicinal and therapeutic potential of Sea buckthorn (Hippophae rhamnoides L.). *Journal of Ethnopharmacology, 138 (*2), 268-278.

Bao, M., & Lou, Y. (2006). Flavonoids from seabuckthorn protect endothelial cells (EA.hy926) from oxidized low-density lipoprotein induced injuries via regulation of LOX-1 and eNOS expression. *Journal of Cardiovascular Pharmacology, 48 (*1), 834-841.

Griel, A. E., Cao, Y., Bagshaw, D. D., Cifelli, A. M., Holub, B., & Kris-Etherton, P. M. (2008). A macadamia nut-rich diet reduces total and LDL-cholesterol in mildly hypercholesterolemic men and women. *The Journal of Nutrition, 138 (*4), 761-767.

Tiano, L., Belardinelli, R., Carnevali, P., Principi, F., Seddaiu, G., & Littarru, G. P. (2007). Effect of coenzyme Q10 administration on endothelial function and extracellular superoxide dismutase in patients with ischaemic heart disease: A double-blind, randomized controlled study. *European Heart Journal, 28 (*18), 2249-2255.

Life Extension. (n.d.). *Atherosclerosis and cardiovascular disease.* Retrieved from http://www.lef.org/protocols/heart_circulatory/coronary_artery_disease_atherosclerosis_01.htm

Hamilton, S. J., Chew, G. T., & Watts, G. F. (2009). Coenzyme Q10 improves endothelial dysfunction in statin-treated type 2 diabetic patients. *Diabetes Care, 32 (*5), 810-812.

Zeb, I., Ahmadi, N., Nasir, K., Kadakia, J., Larijani, V. N., Flores, F., ... Budoff, M. J. (2012). Aged garlic extract and coenzyme Q10 have favorable effect on inflammatory markers and coronary atherosclerosis progression: A randomized clinical trial. *Journal of Cardiovascular Disease Research, 3 (*3), 185-190.

Gao, L., Mao, Q., Cao, J., Wang, Y., Zhou, X., & Fan, L. (2012). Effects of coenzyme Q10 on vascular endothelial function in humans: A meta-analysis of randomized controlled trials. *Atherosclerosis, 221 (*2), 311-316.

University of Maryland Medical Center. (2011, October 14). *Green tea.* Retrieved from http://umm.edu/health/medical/altmed/herb/green-tea

Talbott, S. M., & Hughes, K. (2007). *The health professional's guide to dietary supplements.* Philadelphia, PA: Lippincott Williams & Wilkins.

Wolfram, S. (2007). Effects of green tea and EGCG on cardiovascular and metabolic health. *Journal of the American College of Nutrition, 26,* 4.

Potenza, M. A., Marasciulo, F. L., Tarquinio, M., Tiravanti, E., Colantuono, G., Federici, A., ... Montagnani, M. (2007). EGCG, a green tea polyphenol, improves endothelial function and insulin sensitivity, reduces blood pressure, and protects against myocardial I/R injury in SHR. *American Journal of Physiology. Endocrinology and Metabolism, 55,* 5.

Hodgson, J. M., & Croft, K. D. (2010). Tea flavonoids and cardiovascular health. *Molecular Aspects of Medicine, 31,* 6, 495-502.

Karim, M., McCormick, K., & Kappagoda, C. T. (2000). Effects of cocoa extracts on endothelium-dependent relaxation. *The Journal of Nutrition, 130.*

Grassi, D., Necozione, S., Lippi, C., Croce, G., Valeri, L., Pasqualetti, P., ... Ferri, C. (2005). Cocoa reduces blood pressure and insulin resistance and improves endothelium-dependent vasodilation in hypertensives. *Hypertension, 46* (2), 398-405.

Faridi, Z., Njike, V. Y., Dutta, S., Ali, A., & Katz, D. L. (2008). Acute dark chocolate and cocoa ingestion and endothelial function: A randomized controlled crossover trial. *The American Journal of Clinical Nutrition, 88* (1), 58-63.

Balzer, J., Rassaf, T., Heiss, C., Kleinbongard, P., Lauer, T., Merx, M., ... Kelm, M. (2008). Sustained benefits in vascular function through flavanol-containing cocoa in medicated diabetic patients: A double-masked, randomized, controlled trial. *Journal of the American College of Cardiology, 51* (22), 2141-2149.

Medline Plus. (2011, August 11). *Chromium.* Retrieved from http://www.nlm.nih.gov/medlineplus/druginfo/natural/932.html

Kiefer, D. (2004). Chromium: An elemental essential to health. *Life Extension Magazine*, August 2004. Retrieved from http://www.lef.org/magazine/mag2004/aug2004_report_chromium_02.htm?source=search&key=chromium%20health%20benefits

Harvard Health Publications. (2007, January). *Chromium supplements: chromium, diabetes, and weight loss.* Retrieved from http://www.health.harvard.edu/press_releases/chromium-supplements

University of Maryland Medical Center. (2011, April 2). *Chromium.* Retrieved from http://umm.edu/health/medical/altmed/supplement/chromium

Rivlin, R. S. (2001). Historical perspective on the use of garlic. *The Journal of Nutrition, 131.*

Benavides, G. A., Squadrito, G. L., Mills, R. W., Patel, H. D., Isbell, T. S., Patel, R. P., ... Kraus, D. W. (2007). Hydrogen sulfide mediates the vaso-activity of garlic. *Proceedings of the National Academy of Sciences, 104* (46), 17977-17982.

Predmore, B. L., Julian, D., & Cardounel, A. J. (2011). Hydrogen sulfide increases nitric oxide production from endothelial cells by an akt-dependent mechanism. *Frontiers in Physiology, 2.*

Chung, L. Y. (2006). The antioxidant properties of garlic compounds: Allyl cysteine, alliin, allicin, and allyl disulfide. *Journal of Medicinal Food, 9* (2), 205-213.

Williams, M. J., Sutherland, W. H., McCormick, M. P., Yeoman, D. J., & de, J. S. A. (2005). Aged garlic extract improves endothelial function in men with coronary artery disease. *Phytotherapy Research 19* (4), 314-319.

Life Extension. (n.d.). *Atherosclerosis and cardiovascular disease.* Retrieved from http://www.lef.org/protocols/heart_circulatory/coronary_artery_disease_atherosclerosis_02.htm

Parker-Pope, T. (2007, October 15). Unlocking the benefits of garlic. Retrieved from well.blogs.nytimes.com/2007/10/15/unlocking-the-benefits-of-garlic/

Conclusion

Ahlemeyer, B., & Krieglstein, J. (2003). Neuroprotective effects of Ginkgo biloba extract. *Cellular and Molecular Life Sciences (CMLS), 60* (9), 1779-1792.

About the Authors

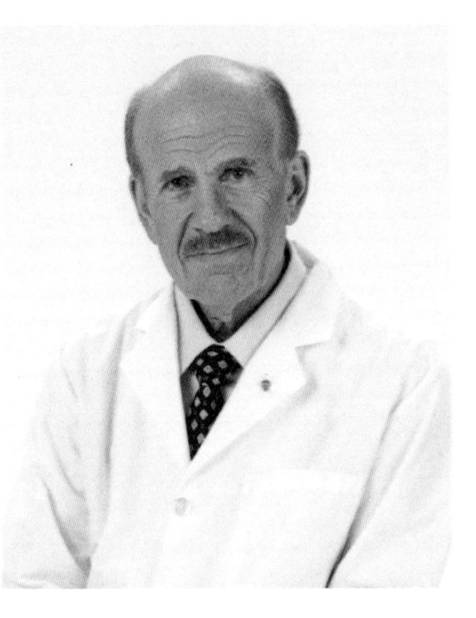

Dr. Louis Ignarro won the Nobel Prize in Physiology or Medicine in 1998, along with Robert F. Furchgott and Ferid Murad, for his research discoveries showing the powerful ability of nitric oxide (NO) to improve cardiovascular health and prevent heart disease. His groundbreaking work—the basis for his 2005 best-selling book, *NO More Heart Disease*—established Dr. Ignarro as perhaps the world's leading authority on nutritional approaches to cardiac wellness, and also led to the development of Viagra. He has spent more than forty years as a research scientist, seeking to understand the incredible role that nitric oxide plays in fostering optimal health. One of his most important discoveries was that antioxidants, along with reducing cell damage from free radicals, increase nitric oxide levels by protecting blood vessel walls—which secrete nitric oxide—from damage.

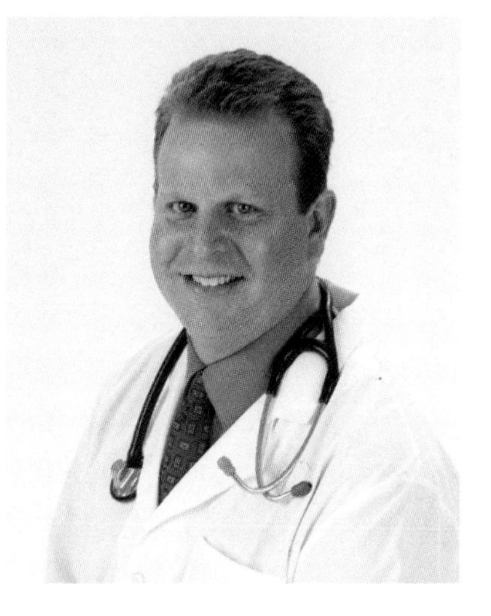

Dr. Andrew Myers is a naturopathic physician who has been in private practice since 1992. As a recognized authority in natural medicines, he is known as one of the world's top experts in the formulation of dietary supplements and their scientific substantiation, as well as in the scientific and clinical validation of natural products. He has formulated and developed hundreds of complete nutritional lines, products, and patents for global brands, including Wal-Mart, Sam's Club, and General Mills. His expertise includes the translation of complicated scientific research into consumer-friendly messaging. Dr. Myers also provides holistic care using natural therapies for the prevention and treatment of cardiovascular disease, cancer, diabetes, and obesity. The founder of Simple Health Value, he is leading the revolution toward simple everyday actions as the foundation of overall health and wellness.

LEARN TO LIVE YOUR LIFE RIGHT

SPREAD THE WEALTH!

Health Is Wealth books are available at quantity discounts for orders of 10 or more copies. Additional volume discounts apply for quantities of 100, 500, or 1000.

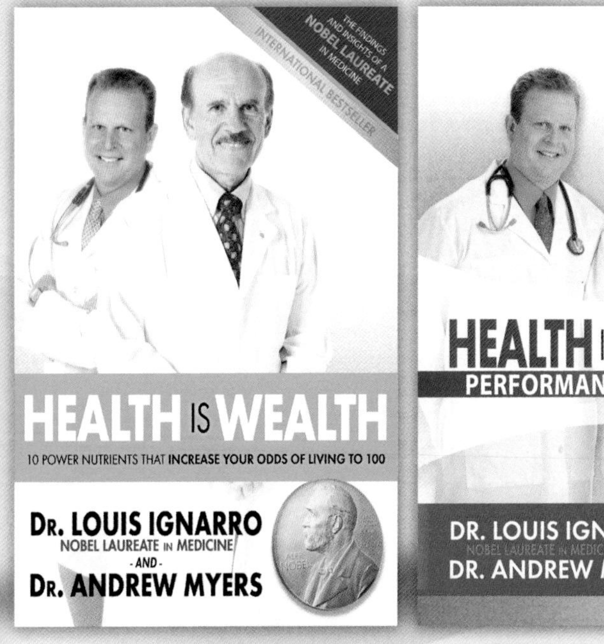

ISBN 978-0-9790229-1-3

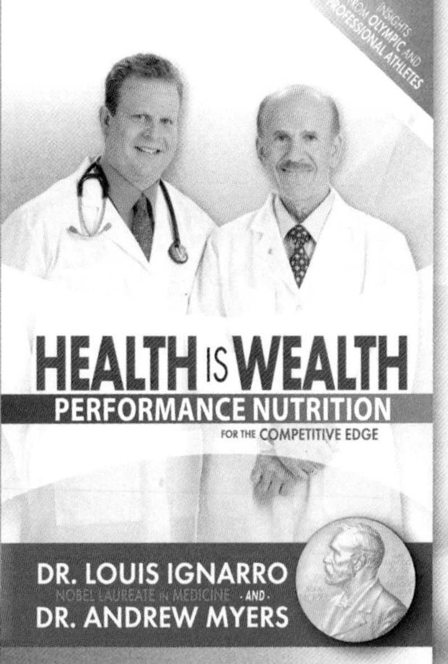

ISBN 978-1-61-389-002-8

To find out about our discounts on orders of 10 or more copies for individuals, corporations, academic use, associations, and organizations, please visit our web site, healthiswealth.net.

LEARN TO LIVE YOUR LIFE RIGHT

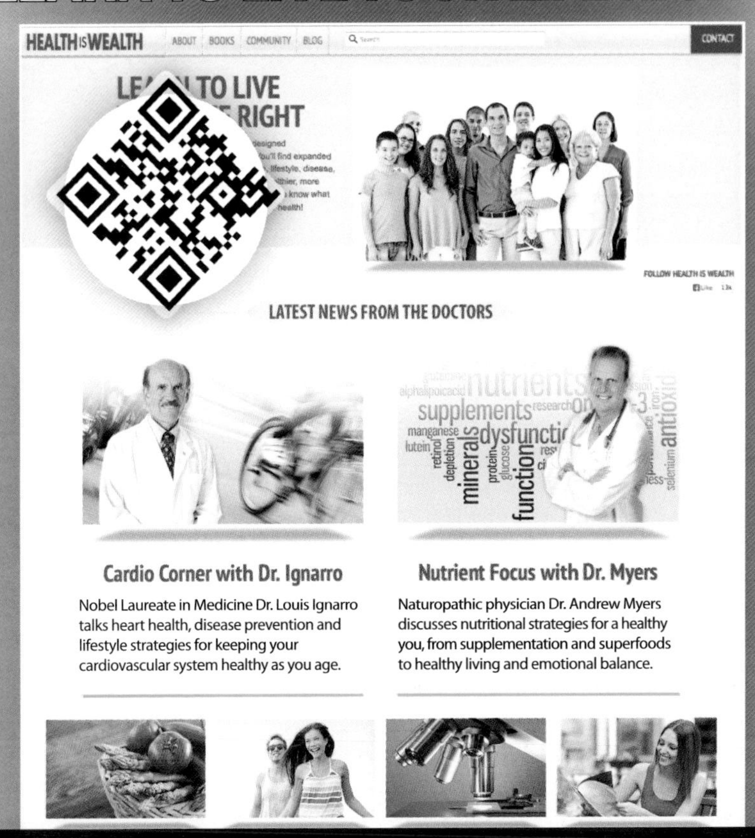

Cardio Corner with Dr. Ignarro

Nobel Laureate in Medicine Dr. Louis Ignarro talks heart health, disease prevention and lifestyle strategies for keeping your cardiovascular system healthy as you age.

Nutrient Focus with Dr. Myers

Naturopathic physician Dr. Andrew Myers discusses nutritional strategies for a healthy you, from supplementation and superfoods to healthy living and emotional balance.

WELCOME TO OUR NEW SITE! We've redesigned **HealthIsWealth.net** with you in mind. You'll find expanded and in-depth content on health, nutrition, lifestyle, disease, and more—all meant to help you live a healthier, more fulfilled life. Enjoy browsing, and please let us know what you think about the content. ***Here's to your health!***

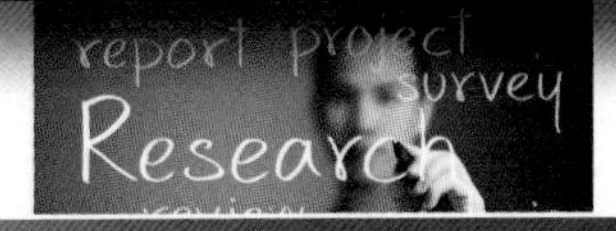

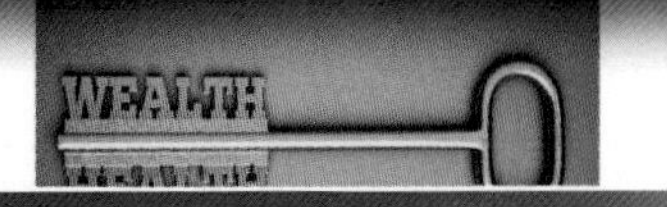

- Read the latest news and blogs from the doctors
- Tell us your Health Is Wealth success stories
- Watch for promotions from Dr. Ignarro
- Get answers to your health questions
- Stay up-to-date on supplement research
- Purchase books and watch free videos
- Follow us on Facebook and Twitter

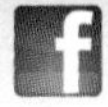
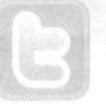